NOTES ON CLINICAL BIOCHEMISTRY

CLINICAL BIOCHEMISTRY

J K Candlish Ph.D
Department of Biochemistry
National University of Singapore
Singapore

M A Crook M.B.B.S, Ph.D, M.R.C.Path
Department of Chemical Pathology
Guy's Hospital
London

World Scientific
Singapore • New Jersey • London • Hong Kong

Published by

World Scientific Publishing Co. Pte. Ltd.

5 Toh Tuck Link, Singapore 596224

USA office: 27 Warren Street, Suite 401-402, Hackensack, NJ 07601

UK office: 57 Shelton Street, Covent Garden, London WC2H 9HE

British Library Cataloguing-in-Publication Data
A catalogue record for this book is available from the British Library.

NOTES ON CLINICAL BIOCHEMISTRY

ISBN-13 978-981-02-1065-6
ISBN-10 981-02-1065-5
ISBN-13 978-981-02-1066-3 (pbk)
ISBN-10 981-02-1066-3 (pbk)

Archaic fevers shake
Our healthy flesh and blood
Plumped in the passing day
And fed with pleasant food.
The fathers' anger and ache
Will not, will not away
And leave the living alone,
But on our careless brows
Faintly their furrows engrave
Like veinings in a stone,
Breathe in the sunny house
Nightmare of blackened bone,
Cellar and choking cave.

EDWIN MUIR

Contents

Introduction

This small book is an attempt to provide a topical gloss* on the basic medical biochemistry course, inevitably perceived by those who are required to partake of it as excessively formula-ridden. Perhaps metabolic pathways are more acceptable than formulae as relevant to later professional practice, but equally, slogging through them is not always inducive to an appreciation of the subject as a real contributor to medicine. Sir George Pickering is said to have remarked that he had not been helped in his management of even a single patient by his knowledge of the Krebs Cycle.** Maybe so, but this distinguished doctor cleverly chose for his disclaimer the pathway in which any defect is almost bound to be fatal *in utero*. Who would disdain a knowledge of glycolysis in treating lactic acidosis, or the urea cycle in an approach to hyperammonaemia?

So it is hoped, then, that if students have access to a fairly slim but stimulating and contemporary text on the uses to which all this biochemistry is eventually put in the clinical years and beyond, they will be able to add to their reading in manner satisfying to themselves and maybe, just as importantly, gratifying to examiners. We hope to demonstrate that you do not need to know a lot of formulae, but that it helps to know some; you do not need familiarity with the fine details of metabolic pathways, but that it is certainly useful to know the gist of a few of the more important ones.

Attempts, in textbooks, to embed basic biochemistry into clinical practice began in earnest about twenty years ago. Thus *A Clinical Companion to Biochemical Studies* by V Schwarz lucidly discussed some cases with a biochemical input, and more recently T M Devlin's *Biochemistry with Clinical Correlations* has become an established, potentially classical treatment which comprehensively covers the massive amounts of material which its title ordains. Here we are not trying to compete with these famous texts, rather trying to partake of their tradition in a way which allows us economically to look at the very latest of the interactions between basic biochemistry and clinical medicine as we go to press in December 1992.

Of course the ultimate clinical application of biochemistry pertains to individual cases. This is however not primarily a case book, although some interesting ones are discussed in relation to adjoining topics when they are illustrative.

We have tried not to circumscribe ourselves geographically – the material herein relates not only to medicine as practised in developed countries; with air travel to exotic places so commonplace, and the growing recognition of electives overseas as part of the medical course, as well as the ethnic admixture around most of today's great city hospitals, nobody can afford to be parochial.

* Gloss   / Scand. origin ... flame, spark / ... **a superficial soft glowing luster or glistening brightness.**
* Gloss   / L. glossa ... a difficult word requiring explanation / ... **an expanded interpretation or commentary.**

Webster's Dictionary

** Quoted with approval from *The British Medical Journal*, 301, 683 (1990) by Professor G Rose, who further emphasises his contempt for biochemistry by misspelling **Sir Hans Krebs'** name.

Note on reference intervals

In the cases discussed in the book reference intervals (normal values) are given for comparison with the patients' results. In modern practice each laboratory is required to determine its own, based on methods and reference populations chosen. The ones quoted here are not to be taken as definitive; however they are consistently used from case to case and they constitute a guide to the reference intervals used in most hospitals.

PART ONE

Structural Patterns and Disease

1a
Muscle Diseases and Proteins

Biochemistry is not very important in establishing the diagnosis of some muscle diseases, but in others it is crucial. By and large muscle diseases can be divided into four categories according to aetiology, thus:

(1) Trauma, e.g. by crushing, drugs and venoms.
(2) Inflammatory, e.g. bacterial and viral infections (myositis).
(3) Metabolic myopathies, e.g. alcoholic and endocrine-based varieties.
(4) Genetically determined, e.g. glycogenoses, Duchenne and Becker dystrophies, malignant hyperpyrexia.

The adult patient with a myopathy will probably present with weakness or wasting, possibly a skin rash (this might be dermatomyositis), whereas a child will have difficulty in rising or walking. Such would be typical of the child who is beginning to develop the symptoms of Duchenne muscular dystrophy, and it is this severe disease for which biochemistry now offers much hope, with the newer knowledge coming in to the clinic itself.

DUCHENNE MUSCULAR DYSTROPHY (DMD)

In some ways the most distressing of the muscle diseases, DMD is an X-linked disorder, thus carried by girls but expressed only in their sons. It usually becomes apparent by about three years of age as retarded motor development, and as it progresses it usually results in the sufferer becoming wheel-chair bound at about the age of twelve, with progressive muscular weakness and premature death, due usually to respiratory insufficiency or pneumonia.

Earlier studies of the serum of DMD patients revealed increases of typical muscle enzymes such as creatine kinase and aldolase, and the estimation of these can still be used to detect cases where the physical signs are equivocal, as well as female carriers of the condition. They cannot be used to detect the condition in the foetus. However, the activities of these enzymes are undoubtedly the consequence of muscle degeneration — that is, they mark the end result of the disease, but do not pinpoint its cause.

The breakthrough into more functionally-related diagnosis came when the gene thought to be responsible for DMD and also the less severe variant called Becker muscular dystrophy, (BMD) was located to band Xp21 of the human X-chromosome by Kunkel. This was done by studying banding patterns in rare patients who showed microscopically visible chromosomal aberrations. He was able to prepare DNA probes complementary to sequences near the gene itself, and to demonstrate heterogeneous deletions. It turned out that the DMD gene is very large, indeed the largest yet discovered in the human genome, extending over at least two million base pairs, with 70 exons. It was not known at this stage what protein the gene might code for, but in the classic example of "reverse genetics", a complementary DNA to the gene was constructed and allowed to express a protein in bacteria. Antisera were raised to this protein, and were found to bind to specific regions in skeletal muscle bearing the sought after natural gene product dystrophin. This is made up of 3685 amino acids and is considered to be in the same family as the structural, cytoskeletal proteins — actinin and spectrin. It is predominantly located at the plasma membrane of the muscle cell, on the inner surface, with a strong relationship with the muscle's transverse tubules, these being linked to the sarcoplasmic reticulum and muscle calcium pathways, important for contraction. It is fairly clear that dystrophin has a structural role anchoring glycoproteins along the muscle myofibrils, although some disagree — it is also found in neuronal tissue taken from the central nervous system, and some claim it is more likely to be involved in calcium flux. Indeed, some 20–30% of affected boys show some mental impairment, indicating that it is too simplistic to view the protein as being entirely involved in muscle contraction.

Patients with the less severe and more slowly progressing BMD variant show an abnormal form of dystrophin in their muscles. This indicates that DMD is caused by frameshift mutations, varying from individual to individual, which however, completely destroy the sense of the coding, whereas in BMD, the mutations are such as not to disrupt the reading frame, and a protein with some sort of biological function is synthesised.

PRACTICAL IMPLICATIONS

How will this new knowledge help you when faced with the DMD problem? There are many different scenarios, and one complicating factor in this disease is that, unusually, frameshift mutations may be both spontaneous and sporadic. However, consider the following situations:

(1) Is a child affected? (for the symptoms may not be entirely clear-cut).
(2) The mother is known to be a carrier (this can often be inferred from pedigree). Is the foetus affected?
(3) Is a girl or wife a carrier?

Biological material is obtained, namely blood from subjects pertaining to situations 1 and 3 (and also as many relatives as possible in the maternal line), but more likely chorionic villi in the context of 2. DNA is prepared from the specimen and incubated with one or more restriction endonucleases, to cut the genomic DNA into a number of large, but unique fragments. These are separated one from another, on the basis of molecular size, by electrophoresis on agarose gels and (Southern) blotted on to a nylon membrane. Meanwhile, X-chromosome probes are made radioactive with ^{32}P and then allowed to hybridise with the restriction fragment length polymorphisms. The specificity of the probes is such that variants in the banding pattern will be seen in those DNA fragments in which mutations have occurred.

Consider a specific case. In this instance, a family sought help in determining whether two daughters were carriers of DMD. A brother had been diagnosed as having the disease on conventional clinical grounds (which would include repeated very high serum creatine kinase activities), but was the first known sufferer in the family. In other words, was this case due to a spontaneous mutation or not? Blood was taken from the two sisters, their brother, and the mother, and treated as above to generate restriction fragment length polymorphisms with one of the available X-chromosome probes (Fig. 1). The mother turned out to be "informative" in that she showed an extra 2.8 kb band which the son had inherited. One of the daughters had only the 1.6 and 1.2 bands, making it unlikely that she was a carrier, but the other (III-2) had the 2.8 kb band. She could have been a carrier, but this was not known for certain, because of the uncertain status of the mother. Despite the banding pattern, which probes only sequences adjacent to the gene, not the DMD gene itself, the mother is only a definite (sometimes called "obligate") carrier if a DMD case is demonstrable in her own parental line, definitely ruling out a spontaneous mutation in the brother. The mother was an only child, and of course her father (now deceased) could not have had DMD since sufferers are assumed not to survive long enough to reproduce. She was questioned closely: could there possibly have been an uncle or great-uncle who died in his teens? Yes, her father had spoken of his brother who died early but she knew little of him; an unmarried elderly aunt, the only other member of that generation, might be able to provide more information. The aunt, fortunately, remembered an elder brother who was unable to walk before his early death.

So the daughter III-2, on discussion with the clinical geneticist (if and when she is old enough) will probably assume that her mother is a carrier, in which case it is almost 100% certain that she is a carrier too.

Although this sort of procedure is a tremendous advance on what went before, it is still not very satisfactory, involving as it does reliance on the knowledge of possible carriers about their forebears. Some laboratories such as those of Thomas Prior are now proceeding to the so-called multiplex polymerase chain reaction (PCR) technique. PCR is explained in Chapter 3a, but essentially involves the

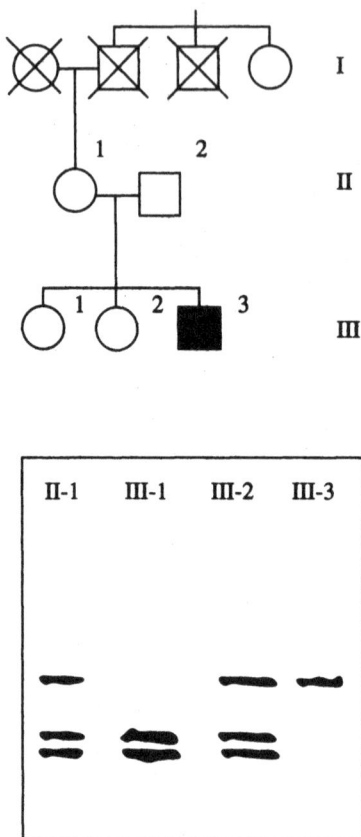

Fig. 1 Tracking muscular dystrophy with the pERT87–15 DNA probe.

Conventionally, squares represent males and circles, females. The deceased are marked with crosses and the known male case represented as a solid square. After electrophoresis of the fragments derived from the genomic DNA of the subjects, the 2.8 kb band in the affected male is found to be present in the mother, although in only one of the sisters, who is almost certainly a carrier if the mother is a carrier. This is still not known for certain unless a case in an earlier generation can be ascertained. (This is a hypothetical case inspired by Ref. 3.)

amplification of specific regions in the genome, using DNA primers (in pairs) to locate the sequences in these regions. Where the base sequence is different from normal, that is mutated, the PCR gives abnormal amplification products, which can be detected on electrophoresis. Since the mutations found so far, though numerous, tend to occur in specific regions of the DMD gene, three separate pairs of primers used in a single PCR reaction can detect 98% of muations.

Footnote

None of the above, you may note, offers any hope for the actual sufferers of the disease — it only indicates ways to establish definite cases and carriers and thus provide genetic counselling as well as selective abortion. Recently, however, it has been reported that normal myoblasts, with appropriate immunosuppression, can be introduced into DMD patients. This is evidently an intermediate step before, hopefully, the normal gene itself can be somatically introduced. Also, bizarrely, a 61-year-old man was recently found to be living a normal life despite lacking almost half the DMD gene. It is speculated that this residual part of the gene codes for that part of the protein binding to the muscle structure; it might also be small enough to be a vehicle for gene replacement therapy, that is the artificial introduction into a tissue of a gene in combination with a virus or some other carrier. Introduction of the gene into dystrophin-deficient mice embryos has already been attempted, with partial success.

Further Reading

1. Turnbull DM and Bindoff L A. Biochemical investigation of muscle disease. *Ann of Clin Biochem* **26** : 472–476, 1989.
2. Kingston H M. DNA analysis of genetic disorders. *Br Med J* **299** : 170–173, 1989.
3. Prior T W, Blasco P A, Doove J L, Leshner R T and Gruemer H D. Use of DNA probes in detecting carriers of Duchenne muscular dystrophy : selected case studies. *Clin Chem* **35** : 679–685, 1989.
4. Prior T W. Genetic analysis of the muscular dystrophy gene. *Arch Pathol and Lab Med* **115** : 984–990, 1991.

1b

Alphafoetoprotein

The glycoprotein with a molecular weight of about 63 000 migrating with the alpha-1-globulins when serum is subjected to electrophoresis, and synthesised by the foetal yolk-sac and liver, was aptly named alphafoetoprotein (AFP) by its early investigators. Although it is generally referred to as though it were a single protein, there is some evidence that its carbohydrate residues depend upon the exact site of synthesis, with the result that AFP may exhibit the phenomenon of molecular heterogeneity. Synthesis by the foetal liver reaches a peak at about thirteen weeks gestation, after which the liver gradually switches to albumin as an alternative product. AFP may thus be regarded as the foetal form of albumin, presumably with analagous functions, although there are some who see it as having a role in the protection of the foetus against immune rejection by the mother, in other words it acts as an immunosuppressant of some sort.

Maternal serum AFP values approximately reflect those of the foetus and can be used to monitor its overall well-being during pregnancy, although this is not often done in practice, there being other and better methods available now, such as high resolution ultrasound.

NEURAL TUBE DEFECTS

If neural tube fusion in the embryo does not successfully take place, then there may be developmental defects of the brain and spinal cord, known as neural tube defects (NTDs). The variety best known to the public is spina bifida, but there is also the rare and even more severe anencephaly, plus others. If these defects render the cerebrospinal fluid "open", that is communicating with the amniotic fluid, then the proteins normally restricted to the foetal body fluids escape to the amniotic fluid and thence to the maternal circulation. This is the basis behind the monitoring of AFP in the mother's blood proteins at about the 16th week of pregnancy. If it is very high then there is a presumption of a NTD, and an abortion can be contemplated *if a NTD is confirmed.* We put this in italics for there are many qualifications and traps for the unwary. For a start, it is important to be sure of gestational age, for the reference values (normal values) against which you presume a rise in AFP are exquisitely dependent upon this. When an international study was done to determine the efficacy of maternal serum AFP measurements in antenatal screening for NTDs, it was found that none of the conventional methods of producing reference intervals — working out means and standard deviations, using curve smoothing procedures to eliminate outlying values and sub-populations — could be applied to the data from each of the 19 centres all over the world. The organisers therefore expressed their values as multiples of the median (MOMs), the median being the most frequent result occurring in a series of measurements. It is less sensitive to outliers than the mean. That is why, almost alone in laboratory reports, you will receive AFP results as MOMs.

In addition to the problems of reference intervals, raised levels of AFP are possible, and therefore may be confusing, in dual or multiple pregnancies, and in threatened abortion and intrauterine foetal death. So confirmatory and exclusionary tests have to be conducted, and these include amniotic fluid AFP, rather than maternal serum AFP. This requires amniocentesis, which in itself carries some risk to the pregnancy , but furthermore amniotic fluid AFP can also be raised in non-neural tube conditions such as foetal oesophageal and duodenal atresia, exophthalmos, foetal nephrotic syndrome and Turner's syndrome, among others. On a practical note, if there is "a bloody tap", that is amniotic fluid contaminated with blood, spurious results may ensue. In the face of all this, another protein/enzyme can be estimated in amniotic fluid — this is a neuronal variant of acetylcholinesterase, which may directly escape from the "open" spinal cord. Diagnostic ultrasound can also be tried. It is on the basis of this battery of tests that the obstetrician may put to the mother the probability of a baby with a neural tube defect.

AFP AND CANCER

AFP has been found to be useful in monitoring primary hepatocellular carcinoma and also hepatoblastoma. There is the slight (but usual) problem of specificity, as other malignancies such as those of the upper intestinal tract and secondary metastases of the liver can also raise it. However, if serum AFP is measured serially, that is repeated over a reasonable period of time, it can be used to monitor tumour progression and thus serve a useful role in management (as opposed to diagnosis) provided that one is aware that non-malignant disease of the liver, for example cirrhosis and hepatitis, can also raise serum AFP, though generally not to the same extent. Fig. 2 shows a patient progression chart in which this concept was used.

Another group of malignancies that AFP measurements have been applied to are the germ cell tumours. Again, serum AFP can be used as a marker for the response of the tumour to chemotherapy regimens, when a decrease in serum levels implies a reduction in tumour mass, as opposed to an increase suggesting relapse. Tumours

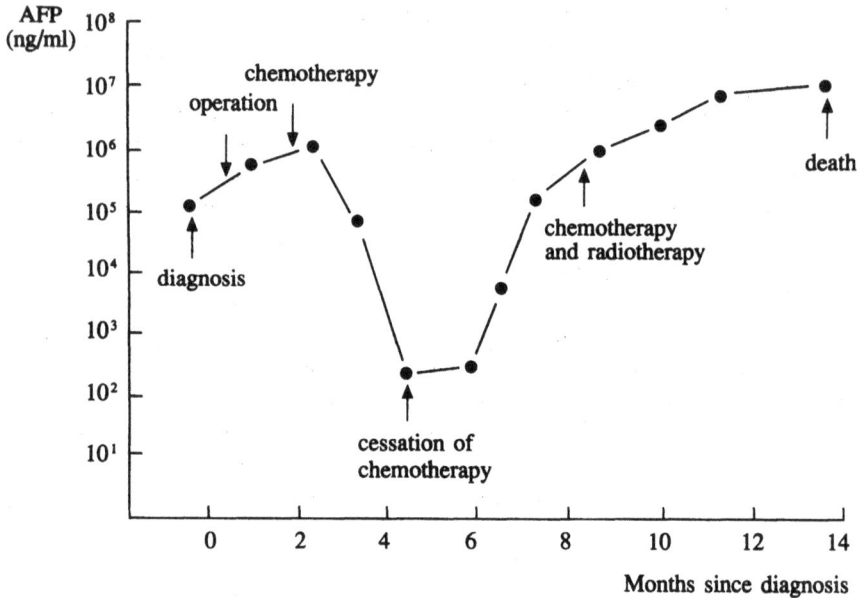

Fig. 2 AFP determinations in the course of treatment for malignant teratoma (tumour containing cells corresponding to all three primary germ layers). Note log scale for AFP.

that have been monitored in this way include gonadal teratomas, and some endodermal sinus and extragonadal tumours. It is said that patients with testicular seminomas do not have a raised AFP and in these cases the protein human chorionic gonadotrophin will be a better tumour marker. Why some tumours express AFP in large quantities is unclear, but it has been suggested that either the tumour cells are more "primitive" in some sense and thus exhibit foetal antigens and foetal products, or the tumour cells lack the means of gene repression control at the genetic level and subsequently synthesise proteins that would normally be suppressed in the adult cell.

AFP AND DOWN'S SYNDROME

Mongolism, or Down's syndrome, or trisomy 21, is well known to be commoner in babies born to older mothers; thus it has been calculated that a mother aged 20 years has a 1 in 2000 chance of producing a baby with the defect, whereas in a mother of 35–40 the risk rises to 1 in 280. When these odds became generally known, it was proposed to reduce the number of Down's babies born by offering amniocentesis and subsequent chromosome culture (which detects the extra 21 member) to all gravidae over 35. This of course conceals a profound fallacy — since there are always many more younger than older mothers, more Down's babies will be produced by the former, and limiting, by whatever means, the number born to the latter group will not effect any substantial reduction. It is therefore very desirable to develop a screening test for younger mothers to identify those who are at risk for Down's babies; in a theoretical way, this should be designed to detect those in whom the risk is at least 1 in 280, so that they can be offered amniocentesis as for the older mothers. It turns out that AFP is useful in this context too, for it is *lowered* in maternal blood when a Down's foetus is being carried. The reason for this remains obscure, but one suggestion is that such foetuses have less efficient yolk sacs and livers in respect of protein production. However, at this point the usual problems intervene — AFP is low in a number of other situations and conditions, such as maternal overweight and diabetes mellitus, and non-viable pregnancy (foetal well-being, as mentioned in the second paragraph above.) Fortunately, a high maternal human chorionic gonadotrophin (HCG) and a low unconjugated oestriol are also markers for trisomy 21. Estimating all three markers increases discrimination and, combined with ultrasound, can allow the obstetrician to calculate which mothers should have amniocentesis, to increase the true detection rate and decrease the number of negative (and therefore, in the end, unnecessary) chromosome cultures.

Summary

We have shown how a biochemical test may be extremely useful clinically, at the same time how much the clinician must be aware of its limitations. It seems at first sight that raised AFP applies to too many different types of patients, and to too many different conditions. In practice though, the patients are largely partitioned before the test is applied; thus pregnant mothers obviously stand in a class of their own as regards the interpretation of AFP results in relation to NTDs, and in men possible seminomas do not generally coincide with potential hepatomas, who may have a history of hepatitis. Or, to put it bluntly, no doctor is going to confuse young mothers with elderly men. So it is not so non-specific in practice.

Further Reading

1. UK Collaborative study: alphafoetoprotein in relation to neural tube defects. *Lancet i*, 1323, 1977. (Although done almost fifteen years ago, this study and its report is a model of clarity and logic in relation to the development of a screening test.)
2. Macrae A R, et al. Position paper: screening for high risk pregnancies with maternal serum alpha-fetoprotein. *Clin Biochem* **23** : 469–476, 1990.

3. Cunningham F G and Gilstrap L C. Maternal serum alpha-fetoprotein screening. *New Eng J Med* **325** : 55–56, 1991.

1c
Tumour Markers

The nature of cancer itself is a matter for more learned works; here we are concerned with the role of biochemistry, and the clinical laboratory, in locating and staging tumours so that appropriate action may be taken by the oncologist. It is obvious that if a tumour arises from the metaplasia of a secretory cell, there is a good chance of pinpointing it by detecting increased secretory product, especially if the product has a well-known function or activity. For example a tumour of the interstitial or Leydig cells of the testis in a prepubertal boy causes virilisation and sexual precocity, and will be marked by excess circulating androgens. From the biochemical point of view, the difficulty is that secretion of the hormones in question tends to be episodic, so that they or their metabolites are often best measured in a twenty-four hour urine specimen. The lymphomas perhaps present a simpler situation since the circulating paraproteins point to the tissue location of the tumour, although of course the differential diagnosis must still be made. But as knowledge of biochemical oncology grew, it was realised that many other tumours fail to synthesise or secrete a conveniently detectable product. Thus hepatomas provide no marker which excludes either other liver diseases or extrahepatic tumours. We need to be able to identify, in the circulation, specific substances released by these difficult tumours, and there has been an extensive search for the same. There has been partial success, and the substances have all turned out to be enzymes or glycoproteins. The approach was to try to identify monoclonal antibodies to extracts of excised tumours, and since the antigenic determinant in the marker extracted has often turned out to be the carbohydrate moiety of the glycoprotein, the newer markers are often named "CA-", standing for "carbohydrate antigen", with a serial number. Tumour markers represent an important topic in biochemical medicine, but it is difficult at the moment to discern any unifying theme, and one has perforce to work through them piecemeal, perhaps leaving out some which have little established importance.

The archetypal tumour marker is perhaps carcinoembryonic antigen (CEA), which is not in itself a single entity, rather a family of related glycoproteins. It was discovered by injecting an extract of human colon carcinoma into rabbits, and demonstrating the presence of this hitherto unknown antigen. It was thought at first to be exclusive to the gastrointestinal tract, but as the detectability of analyses for it improved, in other words, lower and lower concentrations could be detected, it was found in serum of patients with other malignant conditions, and even in normal serum. This tends to be the pattern for tumour markers. Still, laboratories see the number of requests for their analysis increasing year by year, and for a large number of different cancers, as follows.

GASTROINTESTINAL CANCERS

CA 19-9 is the best known of the new glycoprotein markers; it is related to a blood group substance and found in a variety of body fluids. It is high in a majority of patients with advanced exocrine pancreatic adenoma, colorectal cancer, and gastric carcinomas, and also in a minority of those patients who have been newly diagnosed as having these cancers. Here is the crux of the problem. If the markers only detect the disease at an advanced stage, then probably little can be done to help the patient. This is particularly true with respect to the pancreatic adenomas, for which there is no effective treatment. But the tumour marker comes into its own when the growth has been detected by some other method, magnetic resonance imaging perhaps, and it can be used to monitor the efficacy of whatever treatment, perhaps including surgery, has been devised. In the case of gastrointestinal cancers however, postoperative monitoring is just as well carried out with the more established CEA.

CA-50 and CA-195 are other, newer markers for gastrointestinal cancers. The former is elevated in a greater range of non-gastrointestinal cancers than is CA19-9. CA 195 is similar to CA 19-9.

OVARIAN CANCER

Older markers for ovarian cancer include CEA, AFP and HCG, but the newer CA-125 is found in the blood in the majority of patients with an established tumour; again its titre correlates with disease progression. The pattern of marker appearance depends on the exact origin of the tumour however, whether it is mucinous, epithelial or germ cell.

BREAST CANCER

CEA is the long established marker for the prognosis of patients with breast cancer, but CA 15-3 is an up and coming rival. It has some relationship to milk fat globulin and elevated levels are found in 70% of patients with metastases. Early recurrent disease is associated with the absence of oestrogen receptors (ERs) in extracts of tumour cytosol. While only about 30% of an unselected metastatic breast cancer population responds to oestrogen therapy, the response rate doubles if the therapy is targetted towards individuals in which high levels of receptor can be demonstrated in the original growth.

PROSTATIC CANCER

The classical marker of prostatic carcimoma is the enzyme acid phosphatase. It is produced by other tissues but the prostatic isoenzyme can be estimated separately on the basis of differential inhibition or by specific antibodies. It is generally not raised when the growth is still confined to the capsule, but metastasis makes it readily detectable in the serum. Prostate specific antigen (PSA) is a newcomer in this context, being a protein (technically, it is an enzyme too, a serine protease) specific to the prostate. It appears to have some advantages over PAP in terms of sensitivity (detection of true positives).

TESTICULAR CANCERS

Human chronic gonadotrophin (HCG) and AFP are markers for non-seminoma cancers of the testis. The former is raised in some seminoma cases but a better marker is the variant of alkaline phosphatase known as placental alkaline phosphatase (PLAP) named after the site of its initial isolation. One complication is that smoking also raises it.

LUNG CANCER

Only very recently a protein originally isolated from human cervical squamous carcinoma called TA-4 was found to be elevated in the serum of a majority of patients with squamous lung cancer. On the other hand, the enzyme neurone specific enolase (NSE) is raised in small cell carcinoma of the lung.

Summary

There is a fairly clear message; biochemistry has failed to make much progress in the detection of specific markers for tumours in particular organs or cells, especially when such growths are at an early stage and most amenable to therapy. As Dr Weinkove put it, the present set of tumour markers are "late messengers of doom"; those found so far, however, are extremely useful in monitoring progress of therapy or possible recurrence. Examples of this sort of use, in patient progression charts, are given in Fig. 3.

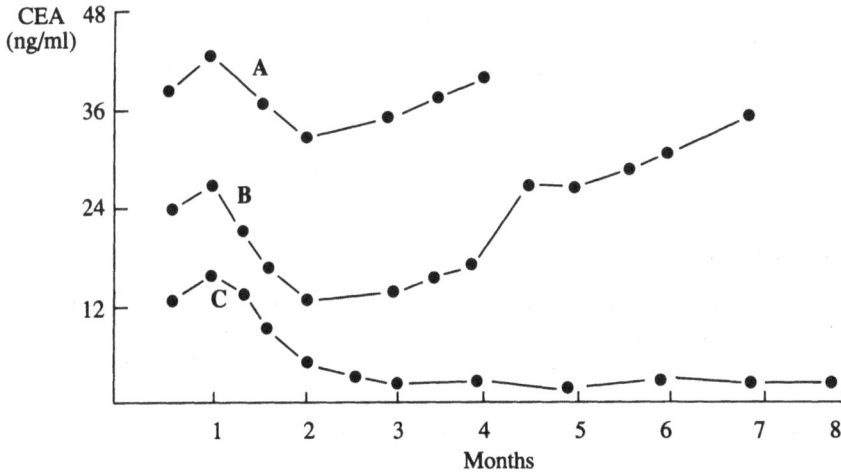

Fig. 3 The use of CEA to chart patient progress.

The three patients were discovered to have liver cancer at about the same time and were treated as soon as possible. Patient A had advanced cancer, showed resistance to chemotherapy as shown by rising CEA after an initial drop, and died four months later. Patient B was operated upon; this seemed to be successful as the CEA diminished but the tumour and/or metastases progressed and he later died. Patient C had successful surgery; serum CEA dropped immediately and was still low 8 months later.

It must be emphasisied again though that many **secretory** tumours, in contrast to the ones discussed above, are recognisable by their products, and tend to be forgotten in any discussion of tumour markers; these are often endocrine, for example phaeochromocytoma with its ultimate product vannilylmandelic acid accumulating in the urine. Also, it is obvious that one has to know a great deal, for interpretative purposes, about the possible cellular origin of cancers from particular organs or tissues, the area of expertise of the histopathologist. A summary of the markers mentioned above is in Table 1.

Table 1   Cancer Markers: the Present Menu

Cancer	Markers			
Breast	CEA	CA15-3	ERs	
Gastrointestinal	CEA	CA19-9	CA-50	CA195
Liver	CEA	AFP		
Lung	NSE	TA-4		
Ovarian	CA-125	PLAP		
Prostate	AP	PSA		
Testicular	AFP	HCG	PLAP	

Note: The abbreviations are spelt out in the text.

Further Reading

1. Sell S. Cancer markers of the 1990s. *Clin in Lab Med* **10** : 1–23, 1990.
2. Beastall G H, Cook B, Rustin GJS and Jennings J. A review of the role of established tumour markers. *Ann of Clin Biochem* **28** : 5–18, 1991.

1d

Cannibals, Mad Sheep and Prions

TRANSMISSIBLE DEMENTIAS

There is a group of dementias, (meaning, broadly, some global deterioration in brain function) that can be passed from a sufferer to someone who subsequently develops the syndrome, in other words, there is a possible transmissible agent involved. They are rare (or so far have been thought to be), of subacute onset and usually fatal. The brain shows neuronal loss, spongiform vacuolation and in some cases extraneuronal deposits of insoluble proteins called amyloid plaques. Debate centres on whether they represent a single disease entity, or can be rationally classified according to the animal (for animals can have dementias too) as well as the exact pathophysiology in man. Some of the names bandied around so far are as follows.

SCRAPIE

This is a degenerative neurological disease of sheep and goats thought to be transmitted by the ingestion of infected placentas. There is some opinion that it is not however a contagious disease under normal conditions of animal husbandry. It has parallels in yet other animals, e.g. transmissible mink encephalopathy. Despite an intensive hunt for the infective agent, it has not yet been isolated; it cannot be cultured by any known method, it does not elicit any detectable antibody, and it is too small to be visualised by electron microscopy.

BOVINE SPONGIFORM ENCEPHALOPATHY (BSE)

BSE or "mad cow disease" aroused a real furore in the middle of 1990. It was thought to be transmitted to cows by feeding them contaminated sheep offal, including inevitably some nervous tissue, with the result that the meat might become potentially dangerous to man. Several continental countries banned British beef, setting off darkly nationalistic sentiments in the tabloid newspapers, and Professor Lacey went so far as to tell a Parliamentary Select Committee that if something were not done we could "lose a whole generation" (of the human population). The Minister of Agriculture however summoned the press to photograph his children eating (presumably British) beefburgers. An interesting politico-scientific dimension surfaced in 1992 when a large consignment of British beef sent to help the deteriorating food situation of the Russians was rejected by them on the grounds that it might carry BSE. As might be imagined, this raised considerable ire among the donors.

Since the incubation period in cattle is about 2–8 years, there was an inevitable delay between the transmission of the agent from sheep, if that was what occurred, and the overt symptoms. In the early eighties, it appears, offal was less exhaustively extracted with organic solvents to produce fat, the market for which had declined, and was also sterilised less rigorously. Cows of course are herbivores, but there is evidence that farmers have persuaded them to eat some sheep material for centuries past, without any manifestation of BSE. The strenuous precautions taken by the

British government (banning ruminant-derived protein in cattle feeds, slaughtering animals suspected of having BSE) were therefore based only on a presumption.

KURU

This condition derives from the former habit, among the Fore tribe of Papua New Guinea, of eating the brains of their deceased relatives. According to Marvin Harris, the writer on food habits, cannibalism of relatives (as opposed to fallen warriors) is seldom practised among premodern groups since it would generate suspicion of eagerness to accelerate demise in the interests of a good meal. However he believes that among the Fore this was outweighed by the stress of protein calorie malnutrition. It had always been traditional to bury deceased members of the tribe in a shallow grave and then exhume the corpse to clean flesh from the bones, without however eating any of it. In the 1920s, the women, possibly because they began to get less meat from their menfolk, exhumed the bodies earlier and ate the brains. Some decades later, the Fore attracted interest among medical anthroplogists for their "laughing disease" or kuru, with its ataxia and dementia. Gajdusek who investigated it in 1967 attributed it to a "slow virus".

JAKOB-CREUTZFELDT DISEASE (JCD)

This condition is a pre-senile dementia which unfortunately has been produced in young people receiving human growth hormone injections prepared from pituitary glands. The hormone is alternatively manufactured in yeast by recombinant DNA technology but preparations laboriously derived from human brains (for it takes hundreds of pituitaries to provide even a single dose) must have carried over some material from undiagnosed JCD subjects. There is a variant of JCD called Gerstmann-Straussler syndrome which is usually familial.

There has been much debate about the scale of these diseases in populations, for most of those who die of dementias do not go to necropsy. Some research groups however do postmortem examinations of samples of patients dying from demential conditions and the workers in St Mary's hospital estimate that about 50% have had Alzheimer's and about 2% have had something very similar, at any rate, to JCD. This would extrapolate to 1500 cases a year in UK as opposed to the 30–40 definitely diagnosed ones. The difference is food for thought!

THE PRION

What is the common factor? Studies have revealed that such infectivity is resistant to nucleases, suggesting an agent devoid of nucleic acid (necessarily present in

viruses). On the other hand, the transmission is blocked by protein denaturing procedures suggesting that the infective agent is a *proteinaceous in*fectious particle or
prion (not, despite the name, a subterrestial space invader). In autopsy brains from
cases of transmissible dementias, a particular protein has been found, called PrP 33-
35sc . It is a posttranslationally modified form of a normal brain protein PrP 33-35c.
The PrP 33-35sc protein principally differs from PrP 33-35c in that it is resistant to
proteinase-K digestion, the normal cellular isoform being completely digested while
PrP 33-35sc is cleaved to form the smaller protein PrP 27-30. This digestion product
is strongly associated with infectivity and has been termed the prion protein (Fig.
4).

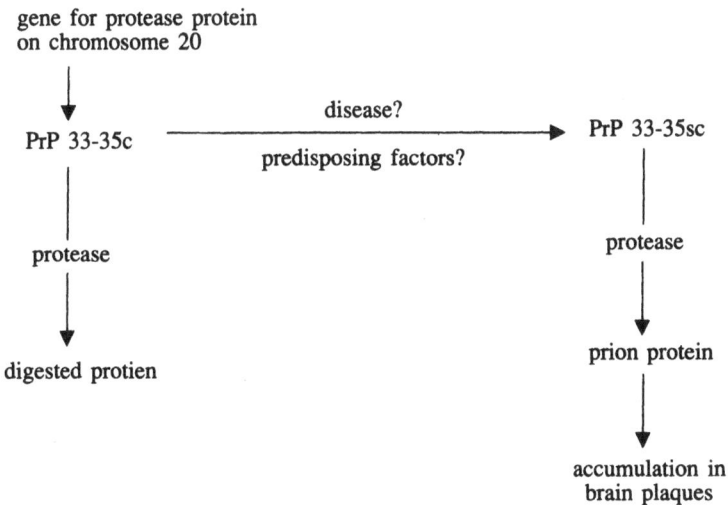

Fig. 4 Postulated formation of prion protein and its involvement in plaque formation in the
brain.

The big question is: what elicits the posttranslational change between the normal
isoform PrP 33-35c and the disease associated isoform PrP 33-35sc? Particularly
important in this context is whether exogenous PrP 33-35sc initiates this transformation, in other words is it in some way autocatalytic of its own replication, or
are other endogenous processes at work? What part could an infective agent play?
Certainly it is known that the PrP gene is located on the short arm of chromosome
20 in humans and it is possible that an abnormality here may predispose the protein
to posttranslational changes.

As to the pathogenesis of the dementia, it has been shown that PrP 27-30 and PrP

33-35sc have the ability to aggregate forming polymers, similar if not identical to fibrils observed in scrapie-infected brains. From immunohistochemical studies involving antibodies raised to prion proteins, cross-reaction has been observed with some cases of amyloid plaques present in the brains of sufferers of the transmissible dementias. The presence of such protein fibrils and plaques may thus contribute to the impairment in brain function. The posttranslational modifications seen in some of these proteins consist of proteolysis and glycosylation which probably result in impaired clearance of the proteins and possible subsequent build-up in the brain.

All this may have relevance to the more common dementias, such as Alzheimer's disease, again a presenile dementia. Some similarities in brain histochemistry between Alzheimer and transmissible dementias have been reported although the evidence for any transmission of the former is weak. Indeed, although deposition of amyloid has been observed in the brains of Alzheimer's disease and also Down's syndrome (trisomy 21) subjects, the amyloid structure is different and the major protein product is coded for by a gene on chromosome 21.

Although the physiological function of the prion protein remains unknown, related studies have helped to elucidate some of the important aetiological and biochemical parameters of the dementias. Certainly there seems to be some good data suggesting a role of prions in some of the transmissible dementias although extrapolation to other dementias would at present be premature, particularly as some undoubtedly have a multifactorial aetiology. Nevertheless, some important clues are now emerging regarding these important medical and social conditions, which may lead to some beneficial therapeutic intervention. Also of interest would be the involvement of prions in other disease states as yet searching for an aetiology. The debate will undoubtedly continue as to whether prions are implicated in these transmissible dementias or whether other particles such as viruses or virions are responsible.

PRACTICAL RECOMMENDATIONS

The following seem forthcoming:
  (1) Check that your beefburgers come from a reputable and quality-minded store or fast food outlet.
  (2) Consider prescribing recombinant (i.e. bioengineered) growth hormone for patients needing growth hormone replacement.
  (3) When doing relief work in New Guinea, try not to share brain meals with local inhabitants.
  (4) Watch the developments in Alzheimer's dementia (Chap. 18e) for if you do not see much kuru or JCD in your practice, you will certainly see plenty of Alzheimer's, and not necessarily only during working hours.

Further Reading

1. Anon. Prion disease — spongiform encephalopathies unveiled. *Lancet* **336** : 21–22, 1990.
2. Bruneri M, Silvestrini M C and Pocchiarai M . The scrapie agent and the prion hypothesis. *Trends in Neurological Sciences* **13** : 309–312, 1988.
3. Collee JG. Foodborne illness: bovine spongiform encephalopathy. *Lancet* **336** : 1300–1303, 1990.

2a

Assessement of Diabetes: From Ants to Amadori

"At the turn of the century a physician who thought he knew syphilis had to know almost all of what was then medical science, including cardiology, neurology, dermatology, epidemiology, obstetrics, bacteriology, pathology, etc., so pleiomorphic was the disease. In an analagous fashion, diabetes and its pathogenesis has brought together almost all biomedical science."

— George F Cahill, Jr

NEOGLYCOPROTEINS

Elderly physicians who have worked in the tropics still point out that a rough and ready (and inexpensive) test for diabetes is to put a dish of suspect urine on the ground; ants will come to enjoy a sugary diabetic specimen but will ignore the normals. This is undoubtedly superior to what early diabetologists in Europe had recourse to, namely tasting the urine. Sophistication made a modest entree about a century ago with Benedict's test for reducing sugars, leading eventually to modern day test strips, which are effectively specific glucose sensors, changing colour in proportion to the amount of the sugar present in the test fluid. They cleverly made use of plant and fungal enzymes absorbed on to paper (Fig. 5).

Thus by laboratory investigation to obtain a quantitative measurement using an analyser, or by the testing of urine — or blood — with an enzyme-impregnated strip, a patient's **glycaemic status** can be assessed. However, the result obtained obviously refers only to the specific point in time at which the blood was taken, and diabetes is a chronic disease; in fact, it is more than chronic, rather lifelong. Prolonged hyperglycaemia is thought to be a major determinant of its complications, especially in its insidious attack upon the kidneys. So some way is needed to assess control of blood glucose over a time span of months or years. There are two ways to do this — home testing of blood by the patient himself so that a progress chart may be maintained, or alternatively to try to find some sort of retrospective index, some marker of status over a preceeding period. This latter approach was not

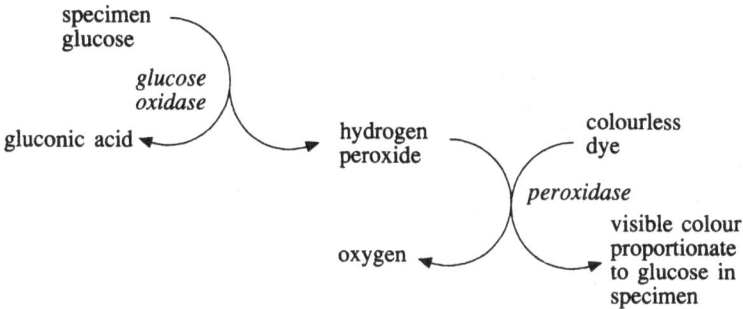

Fig. 5   How glucose is measured on paper strips.
The paper is impregnated with the two enzymes and the dye.

possible until the Iranian biochemist Rahbar noticed that a minor haemoglobin variant was twice as concentrated in the the blood of diabetics as it was in normal individuals. The variant was a fast moving band on the electrophoresis strips he was studying, and had previously been named HbA1c — it was a sub-subfraction of the main human haemoglobin, in other words, the "c" fraction of the type "1" variant of HbA. It turned out be a glycosylated species, that is it has a sugar adduct. (Later the term **glycosylation** fell into disrepute, and the more general terms **glycation**, for the conjugation process was recommended by International Union Pure and Applied Chemistry, who further suggested that the product, HbA1c, should be called a **neoglycoprotein**, specifically, a **neoglycohaemoglobin**). In any case, it was realised that since the life span of the erthryocyte is about 120 days, the concentration of HbA1c is related to the state of glycaemia during this life span. Of course the red blood cells are being synthesised and degraded all the time, so their average age in the blood at any one time is about 60 days, more realistically the period over which measurement of the amount of glycated Hb will give a measure of hyperglycaemia.

HbA1c can be measured in various ways, but perhaps the most visualisable is the high pressure liquid chromatography (HPLC) method, which depends on charge differences among the various species. When glucose reacts with the terminal valines of the beta chains, through an intitial unstable adduct and an Amadori rearrangement, there is the ultimate loss of a charged amino group and HBA1c becomes less positive than HbA (Fig. 6). On this basis, it can be separated from HbA on an HPLC ion-exchange column. On one instrument, the print-out gives a diagram as in Fig. 7. Loading and calculation of the result is automatic so that tens of patient samples can be processed each hour — a very desirable facility when the hospital has a busy diabetic clinic.

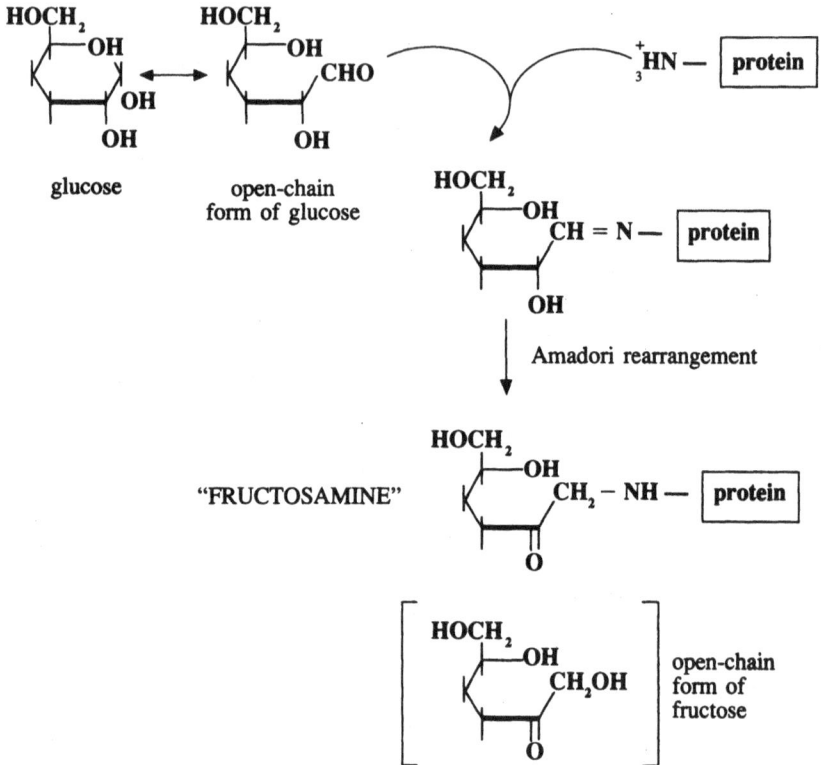

Fig. 6 The protein glycation process.

The lactone form of glucose is in equilibrium with the open-chain form; the latter can form an adduct with free amino groups on proteins. The adduct undergoes a rearrangement involving C1 and C2 of the sugar moiety. This gives it the conformation of the open-chain form of fructose (see structure in brackets), hence "fructosamine." In this scheme some of the irrelevant hydrogens and hydroxyls have been omitted.

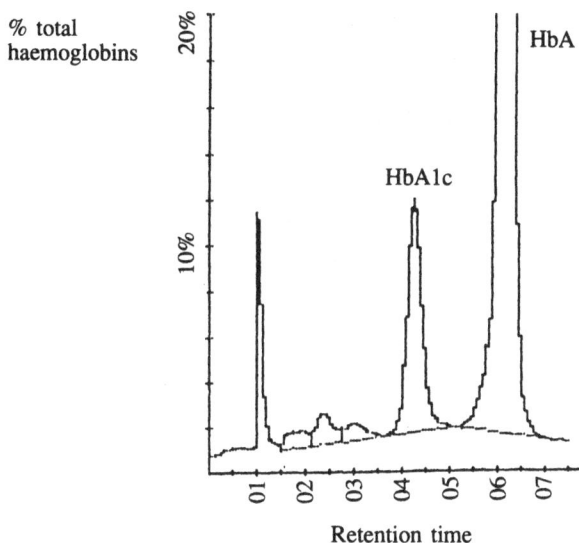

Fig. 7 Separation of haemoglobins on an ion-exchange column.

The HbA1c peak, at a high 11% here, indicates poor glycaemic control. The first peak is a solvent artefact, the next three are respectively the minor glycated fractions HbA1a and HbA1b, and HbF (foetal haemoglobin).

FRUCTOSAMINES

It was realised somewhat later that many other proteins become glycated in the glucose-enriched environment provided by the diabetic body fluids. In the blood serum, the protein in highest concentration is albumin, and the sugar is added to its lysine side chains. Soon it was confirmed that the amount of neoglycoalbumin (often called fructosamine, from the configuration of the sugar after the Amadori arrangement, as in Fig. 6) is raised in diabetics as compared to normal people. Now the maximum life span of albumin molecule is about a month, so the amount of neoglycoalbumin in serum gives an index of glycaemic control in period of about two weeks before the specimen is taken. This would seem to be of inferior utility to the estimation of HbA1c until it is remembered that gestational diabetes is a serious problem, both for the baby and the mother, and that shorter term insight into blood sugar status, perhaps several times within the pregnancy, can be helpful so that appropriate clinical intervention may be undertaken.

Recently, neoglycofibrinogen has been proposed as an even shorter term measure of glucose control. This well-known fibrous protein has a half life of a few days so that its glycated version might provide an index over 2–3 days. It has been argued that the patient's control over weeks or months previously is often not of great interest, but similar information for the previous few days would at least obviate the need for say six to ten fingerpricks for home blood glucose monitoring during that period.

Finally, it is thought that prolonged hyperglycaemia causes glucose adduct formation in many other protein systems.Thus glomerular and capillary basement membranes appear to thicken in diabetics, and this may underly nephropathies and microvascular changes (leading to blindness, for example.) Glycation of myelin sheath proteins may contribute to the neuropathies characteristic of the long-standing disease.

Fig. 8 sums up some of these ideas.

fibrinogen	– 2 days		
albumin	– 2 weeks		used for assessment of glycaemic control
haemoglobin	– 2 months		
basemement membrane	– years (?)		important in pathological processes in e.g. eye and kidney

Fig. 8   Time scales of the various protein glycation processes.

LITTLE WHITE LIES

There is another interesting aspect to the measurement of these neoglycoproteins. Patients naturally like to please their doctors, sometimes by telling them little fibs, such that — if they have insulin-dependent diabetes — then they have been religiously injecting themelves according to the protocol, or if they have the non-insulin dependent type, that they have been taking their medicine regularly, and even sticking to the rather nasty high-fibre diet advised. They may well strive to put on the best presentation for an appointment, behaving themselves in such a way as to make the fasting or random blood sugar on that day seem quite respectable. But the neoglycoproteins, particularly the HbA1c, will yield up the truth!

CASE HISTORY

Let us take an example of how these newer techniques help in patient management. (It is often supposed that biochemistry is primarily concerned with helping **diagnosis**; however, this is not so — most tests are probably concerned more with management and assessment of progress after the diagnosis has been made.) The diagnosis of diabetes is made either on florid signs of the disease (thirst, hunger, loss of weight, perhaps a smell of acetone on the breath) plus a persistently elevated (> 8 mmol/l) fasting blood sugar, or a glucose tolerance test, in which the response to a 75 g dose of glucose at 2 hr is a serum concentration greater than 11 mmol/l. Preferably this should be done twice.

Mr P, aged 55, came back to his clinic in 1988 for a routine check. He had been diagnosed as diabetic some ten years before on the basis of a glucose tolerance test but had no other serious health problems. He was put on tolbutamide at an early stage and then, when medical opinion swung round to the idea of high fibre diets, he was advised to consume appropriate breakfast cereals and brown bread. Later, HbA1c and then fructosamine estimations became available in the referral hospital. He was a taxi driver, behind the wheel for long periods, and although home monitoring with a glucose meter was tried, the doctors did not expect much success under the circumstances. One writes "doctors" because over the years, he saw many different faces across the desk in the clinic, and their owners differed somewhat in testing and management strategies. Table 2 shows a record of his attendances over the years (of course it had to be collated and summarised; patient notes over a ten-year period will never be so compact).

In the last few years the loss of sensation, the steadily rising blood glucose, lipids and blood pressure in Mr P are worrying, although this last has been controlled to some extent by another drug, one of the new calcium channel blockers. He claimed to be doing his best to take the tolbutamide and the later oral hypoglycaemic regularly. But it is the glycated haemoglobin which shows most clearly that, nonetheless, his status is deteriorating. Since he always knows his next appointment it may be that he is jogged into a more assiduous self-management of his medication and diet as it approaches. The fructosamine is not apparently rising as much as the HbA1c which tends to bear out this idea, that he has some success in control over the short term when he really tries. However, fructosamine estimations have been possible only for a few years. The doctor who saw him on 6.2.88 felt that there was no choice but to put him on insulin to avoid real trouble in the ensuing years. An insulin pen is now available and the mechanics of repeated injections are not too horrific; moreover, the pen may now be filled with human insulin, and although there has been an initial scare over human insulin desensitising patients to oncoming hypoglycaemic symptoms, this problem will surely be resolved.

Table 2   Case notes for Mr P (transcription of)

Name: N.P.   Reg. no. 78P00154-E   D. O. B. 3/6/35

Address   6, Moonbeam Avenue, District 10.

Date	Serum glucose (mmol/l)	Urinalysis		Treatment notes
3/4/78	9·4 (f)	ketones −ve sugar −ve		GTT +ve b.p. 140/90 Orinase (tolbutamide) given
12/4/78	11 (r)	ketones −ve sugar −ve		b.p. 145/85
3/5/79	8·6 (f)			attempts at home monitoring unsatisfactory
1/5/80	9·2 (f)	ketones −ve sugar −ve		b.p. 150/95
2/12/81	9·1 (f)			b.p. 150/90
			HbA1c %	
13/5/82	9·9 (f)		7·3	Orinase cancelled glibenclamide prescribed
23/6/83	12.2 (r)		7.1	High fibre diet advised b.p. 150/90
15/5/85	9·5 (f)	ketones −ve sugar −ve	8·3	b.p. 160/95 Cholesterol 6·2 mmol/l
3/4/86	8·8 (f)		10·1	b.p. 180/105 thiazides prescribed
			fructosamine (mmol/l)	
9/8/87	8·6 (f)		14·1 3.1	b.p. 180/110 nifedipine prescribed
10/3/88	9·2 (f)		16.2 3·4	b.p. 160/90 cholesterol 6·9 mmol/l
15/4/88	9·3 (f)	ketones −ve sugar −ve	16.0 3·6	b.p. 160/95 cholesterol 7·9 mmol/l

f = fasting

r = random

END-ORGAN DAMAGE

There are many medical advances which prolong life but which reveal a set of unsuspected pitfalls and problems. The introduction of insulin therapy was a signal example thereof — it enabled Type 1 diabetics to survive, but left them at great risk for a number of grave complications, particularly neuropathies and microangiopathies, the latter manifesting above all in the retinal and glomerular vessels. Thus blindness and kidney failure are ever-present dangers for long-standing diabetics. There is still intense discussion as to whether these phenomena are the result of the glycation of structures like the glomerular basement membrane, or are multifactorial in themselves, but whatever may be their basis, it is very desirable to have a way of detecting the deterioration in patients' microcirculation. In this context, the measurement of albumin in the urine has come up very strongly and currently attracts intense research.

The kidney does not normally filter protein in large amounts, but progressive glomerular angiopathy allows passage of relatively small proteins like serum albumin. It has to be present in substantial amounts in the urine to be detectable by normal methods, however. (By that we mean stick tests like "Albustix" or the dye-based methods on routine clinical chemistry analysers.) To indicate microalbuminuria, the patient's urine must show albumin greater than about 30 mg/24 h, but below the level of persistent gross proteinuria, 250 mg/24 h. To these ends radioimmunoassays with detectabilities down to less than 30 mg/24 h were developed and have found wide applicability.

Two points arise. First of all, proteinuria is also related to hypertension, and blood pressure has to be looked at carefully during the interpretation of results. Secondly, there is an oddity in nomenclature here. Of course, it is not "microalbumin" which is measured, but small ("micro") amounts of albumin. Fortunately, this unfortunate coinage seems to be unique to this area.

Summary

The material set out above well serves to expand one's knowledge of metabolic disorders. It gathers together strands of protein and carbohydrate chemistry learned early in the biochemistry course within the framework of a very important disease (for some say if you know diabetes, you know medicine — such used to be said of syphilis, see the quotation at the head). It has important links with clinical nutrition and with other primary or secondary metabolic derangements such as hypertension, obesity and atherosclerosis.

Further Reading

1. Alberti KGMM. If I had insulin-dependent diabetes. *Br J Clin Practice* **42** : 269–271, 1988.
2. Hammer MR, John PN, Flynn MD and others. Glycated fibrinogen: a new index of glycaemic control. *Ann Clin Biochem* **26** : 58–61, 1989.
3. Cohen MP. *Diabetes and protein glycosylation: measurement and biologic relevance*. New York: Springer Verlag, 1986.
4. Leslie RDG (ed). Diabetes. B*ritish Medical Bulletin* **45**, 1989. (Whole issue.)

2b

Sugar: And Some Honeyed Words

Even those lacking a sweet tooth are liable to be continuously bombarded by sugar, or sucrose, to use the chemical term. From being a luxury available only to the rich (this was before the development of plantations and steel rollers for crushing the cane) it has become readily available to all — more than that, as an unseen additive to foodstuffs we do not generally consider to be sweet, such as soups, hamburgers, and baby cereals — even the "bitter" lemon for mixing with gin. Sucrose is one of the candidates for the opium of the people — easing the pain, it has been suggested, of their traumatic entry into the industrial age. In righteous reaction, it has been blamed for diabetes, dental caries, obesity and heart disease. On the other hand again it has to be recognised that many groups, such as manual workers in heavy industries, and children, may need large and easily assimilable amounts of energy, a role readily filled by sucrose. What is the medical consensus on it however, and on its salient constituent, fructose? Should you ask your patients to cut it out altogether if they wish to slim? Should you suggest fructose for diabetics, or for sobering up after a night on the tiles, and what is the value of sweetening substitutes like honey, saccharin and aspartame? All of these are available without prescription, so the only debarrment to misuse is advice!

HONEY

Until the large-scale production of sucrose by courtesy of tropical agriculture, honey was the only easy way of sweetening foodstuffs. It is largely fructose and glucose (about 30% by weight each), the balance being water (17%), maltose (7%) and sucrose (2%). In the West, it is now largely a breakfast adjunct. Since it is touted as being "natural" the health food shops would like us to buy more of it. They have perhaps unexpected allies in Arab and Moslem medical practitioners, among whom its properties are particularly favoured due to specific commendation in the Koran. Certainly its almost anhydrous nature makes it sterile, and it has been proposed as an unguent for wounds. The antibacterial properties have been supposed to be contained in a substance called inhibine, which may be identical to hydrogen peroxide. Such applications may be useful if you cannot obtain antibiotics, for example, but in view of the very small amounts of constituents other than the two monosaccharides, we await more definitive work on their real benefits.

SUCROSE AND FRUCTOSE METABOLISM

The difference between sucrose/honey and other common carbohydrate foods is their provision of fructose as well as glucose, although recently an additional source of fructose has been the corn-derived syrups favoured by the food industry in that weight for weight they are sweeter than glucose-based syrups.

Although we are familiar with fructose phosphates as components of glycolysis, free fructose in itself is not synthesised by human tissues, with the exception of the seminiferous tubules. Why this oddity? Presumably on introduction to the vaginal and uterine epithelium, which have a vigorous glucose metabolism but less efficient manner of assimilating fructose (due to the absence of fructokinase) the delicate sperm (after all even normal body temperature is too much for them) can be assured of their own private energy supply in the seminal plasma.

Fructose is however extensively utilised by one human tissue, the liver (very small amounts may be taken up by others) for of course it has to deal with the incoming sugar from the diet at first pass. The uptake is not an insulin-dependent process, as for glucose. The first step in metabolism is phosphorylation, yielding fructose 1-phosphate (Fig. 9). The end-products are glucose and lactate (about 70% and 30% respectively under normal circumstances). Administration of fructose by mouth or intravenously (it is occasionally incorporated into total parenteral nutrition fluids) is therefore equivalent to giving these two substances. Note that ATP is required, as is NADH, the reduced form of the coenzyme, and there are in fact multiple pathways possible — the glyceraldehyde 3-phosphate may alternatively be converted to glycerol phosphate as a constituent of triglycerides.

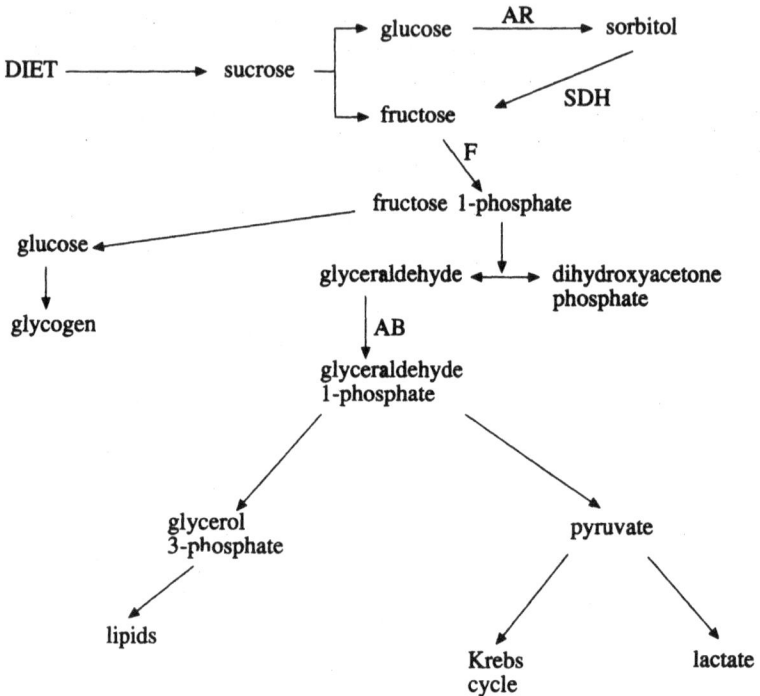

AR – aldose reductase, converting glucose to sorbitol in the eye

SDH – sorbitol dehydrogenase

F – fructokinase, lacking in fructosuria

AB – aldolase B, lacking in fructose intolerance

Fig. 9 Pathways of fructose assimilation.

Depending on the conditions, fructose can yield a wide multiplicity of products, mainly in the liver. Many of the transformations shown consist of multiple steps, and many are reversible; reversibility is however ignored to show the flow of carbon atoms along the various pathways after a bolus of sucrose or fructose is ingested.

SUCROSE, FRUCTOSE AND DIABETES

Many decades of advice to diabetics to eschew carbohydrates were overturned during the 80s, so that now it is recommended that 55–66% of their calories come from this source, as long as there is also adequate fibre. Thus the use of sucrose in the diets of diabetics, traditionally banned due to the perceived risk of aggravating hyperglycaemia, is now acceptable, for several studies showed that it did not result in greater hyperglycaemia than other common carbohydrates. In other words, it is now felt that sucrose may *replace* other sources of energy, not supplement them. This is important, as it has been shown that if calories are in excess, glucose tolerance will certainly be impaired (Fig. 10).

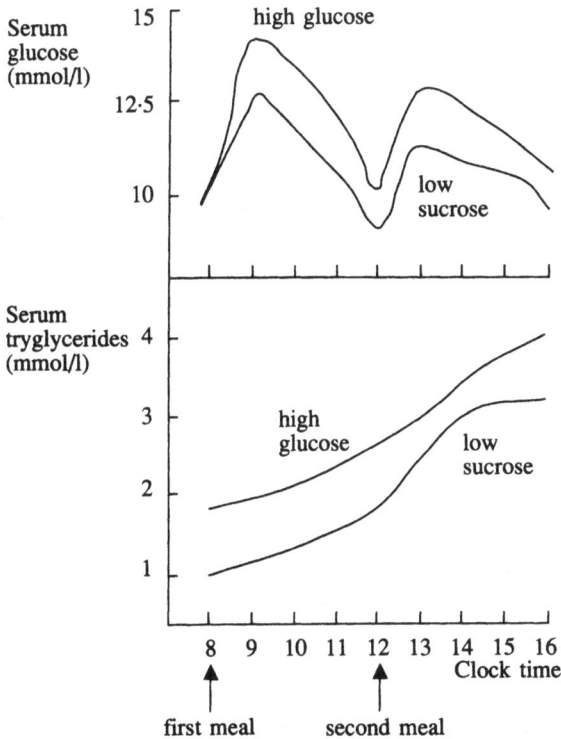

Fig. 10   Effect of dietary sucrose on diabetics.

High and low sucrose diets were given to non-insulin dependent diabetics for two weeks, then during the eight hours over which blood was taken hourly, as shown. Evidently the sucrose affects the postprandial glucose, but has a more permanent effect on serum triglycerides. Based on a report by G M Reaven in *Nutr Rev* **344** : 65–73, 1986.

Because fructose is assimilated in a noninsulin dependent manner it was with strict logic introduced into diabetic diets or snacks, such as "diabetic chocolate" (as has sorbitol, its reduction product, Fig. 9). However deficient insulin production (Type I diabetics) or insulin receptor function (Type II) may be, it should provide a ready source of energy. It has certainly been established that plasma glucose does not increase as much after an acute oral dose of fructose alone as after an equal amount of glucose. We might infer this from the diagram, in that there must be some delay in converting the fructose to glucose, and anyway part of it is diverted to three carbon compounds such as lactate and glycerates. The consensus seems to be that in Type I diabetics, where the pancreas produces no insulin, it is a valuable source of energy. In Type II diabetics the primary aim is said to be weight control, so that total calories should not in any way be augmented by sweeteners.

Fructose and Alcoholic Detoxication

Fructose, when it is rapidly phosphorylated in the liver, is split into trioses and these yield at least a modicum of glycerol or its phosphate. This needs NADH (Fig. 9), which is one of the primary products of alcohol metabolism. So fructose ingestion would seem to be a good way of mopping up NADH and accelerating the detoxication process. Glucose would tend to have the same effect in so far as it is also a precursor of glycerol via the triose phosphates but again, it has to be emphasised, glucose metabolism is dependent upon the rate-limiting effect of insulin. Rapid sobering-up with fructose has not been much of a success in practice, although it can do little harm, except for the danger of hyperuricaemia and perhaps lactic acidosis.

Defects of Fructose Metabolism

There are several inborn errors of fructose metabolism. The rare cases of fructose intolerance are due to absence of the aldolase. There is hypophosphataemia as a conseqence of the irreversible phosphorylation of the ingested dose, and hypoglycaemia due to suppression of glucose release from the liver; apparently this is a direct effect of fructose 1-phosphate on phosphorylase. Moreover its accumulation, or possibly the massive depletion of ATP, seems to damage the liver cells and there is often hepatomegaly, with the sufferer becoming jaundiced. Subjects with the condition learn to avoid sweet foods, and it is said that they do not suffer from dental caries.

Essential fructosuria on the other hand is due to lack of the phosphorylating enzyme fructokinase in the liver, and is harmless despite the large amounts of fructose present in the urine after it has been ingested.

SUGAR, OBESITY AND HEART DISEASE

Although fructose and sucrose are safe for diabetics when taken as replacement calories, there is concern that nonetheless they may be more hyperlipidaemic than other carbohydates, with the implication of an increased risk of heart disease. Unfortunately, there is much controversy on this matter. On the surface, it might seem to be an easy enough matter to feed either fructose or sucrose or glucose to diabetic individuals and see what happens to their blood lipids, but it seems that various populations can react differently within even the simplest experimental protocol.

One reason for this may be that diabetes is in fact a group of diseases, and each observed population will have a different spectrum of underlying pathologies. On the whole, however, scrutiny of the literature reveals that neither sucrose nor fructose is likely to have a profound effect on blood lipids.

Comments

Here the basic glycolysis-linked metabolism of a common sugar has implications in diabetes, inherited diseases of metabolism, fertilisation, alcoholic intoxication and even heart disease. Although these may be largely controversial, it is well worth knowing something about fructose and its metabolism. One can see how central is the glycolysis pathway and how consistently a knowledge of its basic steps and control is repaid. Perhaps the most basic problem, in pactical terms, is balancing the undoubted cariogenic effect of sucrose against the obvious need of children for rapidly assimilable energy. If too much rapidly assimilable energy leads to obesity (Chap. 10b) the dilemma is solved — no sweets!

Further Reading

1. Hallfrisch J. Metabolic effects of dietary fructose. *FASEB Journal* **4** : 2652–2660, 1990.
2. Bantle JP. Clinical aspects of sucrose and fructose metabolism. *Diabetes Care* **12** : 56–61, 1989.

3a

DNA: New Twists to the Helix

"A late twentieth-century Holmes would be glad of his Watson. As a modern medical man, Dr Watson would be well-versed in genetics. He would know how a drop of blood or semen or a hair follicle could — at least in theory — prove that a certain person had been at the scene of a crime ..."

— The Economist, June 24th, 1989

DNA is always full of surprises; one such was the discovery of introns, sequences in the genome which are not expressed, that is they do not code for proteins; indeed the majority of DNA in the human genome appears not to be expressed. It might seem that such regions are less worthy of study, at least as a priority, than the exons, but they have been the basis of some of the most exciting advances in medicine in recent years. The story of how Jeffreys came to capitalise on his expertise in studying them has been told many times now; he was examining non-coding sequences in the myoglobin gene which were highly repeating (the so-called minisatellite regions), the first of which had previously been detected by Wyman and White in 1980. In the myoglobin gene the minisatellite region consists of a 33 base-pair sequence repeated four times in tandem (meaning end-to-end). Such hypervariable regions, of which there may be over 1500 in the human genome, differ from one locus to another and from one individual to another, this freedom being possible, of course, precisely because they are not expressed; expressed sequences or exons have to be similar from one individual to another because they code for specific functional enzymes and proteins). The hypervariability of the minisatellite regions is generated by the number of repeats of the tandem sequences (which is why they are also called **variable number tandem repeats** or VNTRs), but Jeffreys found that they all contain non-variable **core** sequences. (A diagrammatic representation of this quite complicated scenario is attempted in Fig. 11.) Jeffreys constructed DNA probes, that is complementary base sequences, for parts of the core sequence and used established techniques of molecular biology to establish genetic relationships.

The technique, briefly, is to chop up the genomic DNA with a restriction endonuclease, and produce large polynucleotide fragments. These vary in size and sequence according to the number of tandem repeats and the base sequences within the minisatellites, in other words the pattern of fragments will distinguish one individual from another, except for identical twins. The fragments are sorted according to size by electrophoresis on agarose gels, and after Southern blotting to concentrate them on a membrane, are overlaid with the radioactive probe, which binds to the core sequences, revealing a series of bands often, if fancifully, likened to a supermarket bar-code (Fig. 11). Because the DNA in the minisatellite regions of each individual is unique, it will give a unique pattern of bands, but the more closely related the individuals are, the more will their bands correspond. Of course, in the case of identical twins, the bands show complete correspondence.

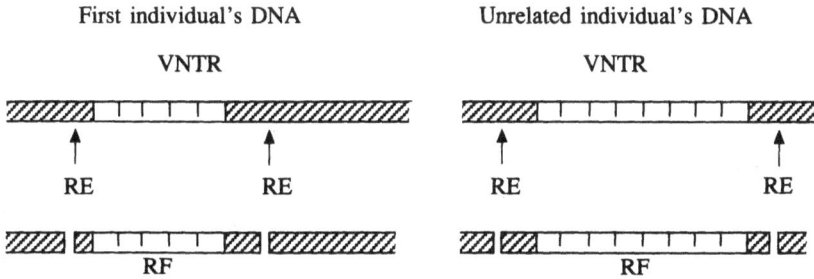

Electrophoresis, blotting and hybridisation; these fragments being from unrelated individuals; being of different molecular weights yield different bands

Fig. 11 The general principle of the DNA fingerprinting technique.

The hypervariable regions (hypervariable because of different numbers of tandem repeats in non-related individuals) are partitioned by endonuclease digestion into restriction fragments of diverse molecular size. These are separated by electrophoresis and detected by complementary DNA probes for the hypervariable regions. Closely related individuals will tend to give similar patterns, unrelated individuals diverse patterns.

VNTR = variable number of tandem repeats
RE = restriction endonuclease
RF = restriction fragment

THE GHANAIAN BOY

The first case, or at least the first widely-publicised one, to which the new technique was applied, was that of the Ghanaian boy who wished to return to Britain after a stay with his father, but was refused entry into the country by the immigration authorities. They disputed the mother's claim that he was genuinely her son. The father was not available for testing, but the individual patterns of restriction fragments ("DNA fingerprints") showed that the mother shared half her DNA pattern with the boy, and half with her other children who all, incidentally, shared the same paternal fragments, showing that they all had the same father. The authorities, namely the Home Office, had no choice but to bow to the evidence.

THE PITCHFORK CASE

Then came the famous rape case in Leicestershire; there had been previous convictions on the basis of DNA fingerprints from semen specimens recovered from victims but the Pitchfork case was sensational. In 1983 a girl was raped and murdered in a Leicestershire village, but the crime remained unsolved. Unfortunately, a similar outrage occurred not half a mile away in 1986. DNA fingerprint evidence from semen proved that the same man had been responsible for both crimes and in the interim also helped to clear a seventeen-year-old youth who had been arrested on suspicion (and had spent a month or two in jail!). But the police were convinced that a local man was responsible and asked all the male inhabitants of the area, between the ages of 13 and 30, to give blood for matching of their leukocyte DNA to that from the semen specimens. Five and a half thousand came forward for testing, but no match could be made in the laboratory. By August 1987, despite over 7000 statements, 25 000 computer entries, and the offer of a £20 000 reward, the police had to concede that they had no leads.

One Colin Pitchfork, however, had failed to attend two appointments with the forensic scientists and persuaded a workmate to impersonate him and give blood under his name on the third occasion. The deception came to light due to the indiscretion of the latter (he was later quite rightly jailed for conspiring to pervert the course of justice) and when Pitchfork was eventually arrested his DNA matched the forensic specimens. He was convicted and sentenced to life imprisonment in January 1988.

THE CASTRO CASE

All seemed well for the technique, which became well accepted by forensic scientists in Europe and in the USA, until the Castro case in New York. A pregnant woman and her child were murdered and Jose Castro, when arrested in connection with the crime, had a spot of blood on his watch which he claimed was his own. The spot was uplifted for matching against the deceased's DNA by the Jeffrey method, performed in this case by a company called Lifecodes Corporation. At a pre-trial Frye hearing to assess the validity of the new identification system (an American judicial technique to avoid blinding the jury with bogus science, as it were) the conclusions from this particular test were strongly challenged by the defence lawyers. Among other things, they objected to a correction made for "band shift" — this is the the phenomenon whereby inconsistencies in the gel cause specimens to run out of alignment even though their bands perhaps correspond to each other. Some of the prosecution witnesses even went over to the defence on mature consideration of the deficiencies in the way the company practised its techniques. So the case was a watershed in the apparently uninterrupted success of molecular genetics. In the end though, the legal authorities could not fault the theory; they insisted merely on proper control, accreditation and training procedures. (By a stroke of supreme irony, Castro eventually pleaded guilty.)

THE POLYMERASE CHAIN REACTION INTERVENES

The DNA fingerprinting technique based entirely on restriction endonucleases, electrophoresis, and probes, salient though it was, was introduced just before another technique which has so revolutionised biology and genetics that it stands in a class of its own, so much so that it enabled DNA fingerprinting to be simplified and speeded up. This is the polymerase chain reaction (PCR). PCR also markedly increases the sensitivity of the fingerprinting technique, sensitivity in this sense meaning the amount of starting material, genomic DNA, which is necessary in order to obtain a meaningful result. Theoretically, it can use as little as one cell, or even one single DNA molecule; this is because it is a process of exponential amplification, as diagrammed in Fig. 12. It is necessary to know specific oligonucleotide sequences flanking VNTRs, which are annealed to the separated DNA strands. When the nucleotides and DNA polymerase are introduced (primer extension phase) the VNTRs are replicated, plus a run-on of unwanted polynucleotide. By the third cycle the final products appear, and it is these that are amplified exponentially thereafter. If it is recalled that they differ from one individual to another in terms of size, the amplified products need only be electrophoresed and visualised to give the differential banding patterns. No restriction endonucleases or radioactive probes are necessary.

In practice, PCR has allowed a further dimension to be added to the fingerprinting procedures. The original technique, as outlined above, sorted individuals on the basis of the number of tandem repeats within the targetted DNA sequence; PCR, because of its capacity for specific amplification, allows the study of mutations

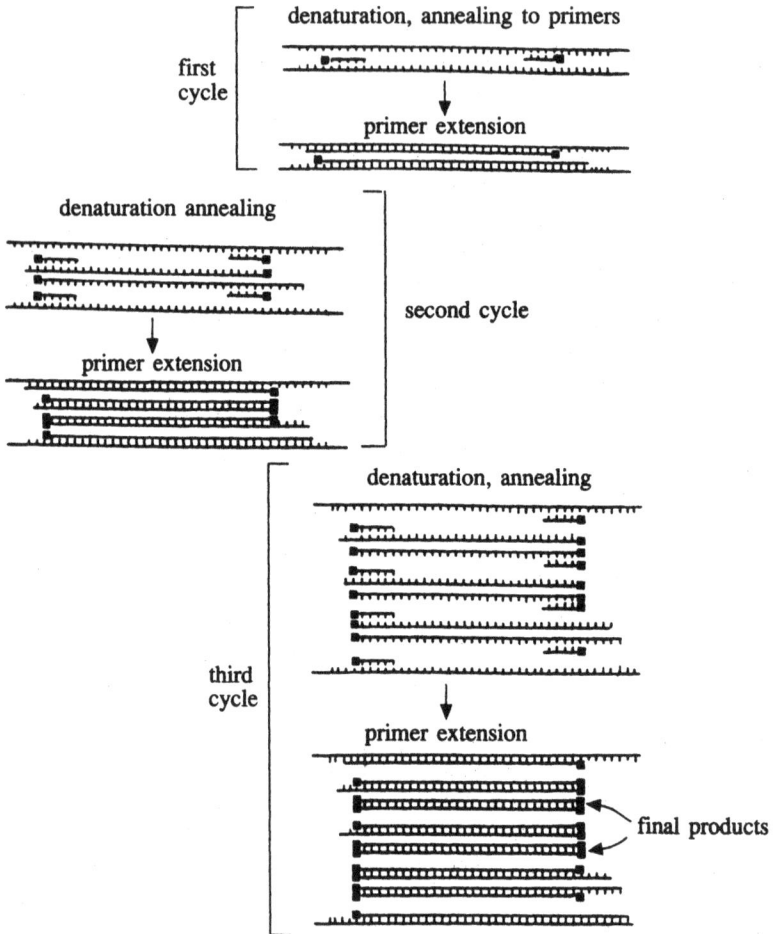

Fig. 12   Principle of the polymerase chain reaction.

Basically, polymerisation can be conducted in one vessel because the DNA polymerase can survive cycles of heating and cooling. Initially the genomic DNA double helix is separated into single strands (shown here as serrated lines) by heating, then cooled and allowed to anneal to DNA primers (the small serrated segments) complementary to the portion of the gene to be amplified. Then the enzyme and the added nucleotides form double-stranded DNA in the primer extension step. In the second cycle there is again denaturation by heating, annealing to primers in the cold, then primer extension. The first segments of DNA of the desired length are obtained, but annealed to strands of indeterminate length. It is only in the third cycle that the final products are obtained, but are thereafter multiplied exponentially. Note also that the base sequence of the gene, or part of it, has to be known for the design of the primers.

within the tandem repeats. The implications of this powerful extension are being worked out.

APPLICATIONS IN MEDICINE

Where are the applications of DNA profiling to medicine, apart from forensic medicine? The applications seem limited only by the imagination of the user. The technique has been used to document the first instance of a woman becoming pregnant by a man with Down's syndrome, for example; this had been thought hitherto to be an unlikely event. In an entirely different context, if buffy coat cells can be identified as those of the donor at various stages after a bone marrow transplant, then they indicate the continuing success of the transplant — they have survived the immune attack of the host. Indeed the origin of any cell can be checked against its putative source, parent, or relative. At the time of writing we await, for example, the results of tests on a skeleton in Brazil, which may show if they derive from the Nazi war criminal Dr Joseph Mengele; only if the fingerprints show that the DNA from the bones sufficiently matches that of his son will the Israeli government close its file.

Bizarrely, even surrealistically in the light of the serious issues above, it has even been suggested that the DNA fingerprinting method be used to detect inheritors of titles (ranging from Scottish clan chiefs to English dukedoms) who might be illegitimate or conceived by artificial insemination, so that they can be prevented from interrupting the true "blood line." The catastrophic nature of this eventuality is not obvious to the plain man in the twentieth century; indeed the mere existence of the controversy suggests that we are still not all living in it.

Further Reading

1. Connor S. Genetic fingers in the forensic pie. *New Scientist,* 28th Jan, 1988, p. 31.
2. Cawood AH. DNA fingerprinting. *Clin Chem* **35** : 1832–1837, 1989.
3. Neufield PJ and Colman N. When science takes the witness stand. *Scientific American* **262** : 18–25, 1990.
4. Farr CJ and Goodfellow PN. New variations on the theme. *Nature* **354** : 184, 1991.

3b

The Modern Day Plague

"After 28 years of blameless and by many people's standards (but not mine) dull heterosexual monogamy, I visited an African medical school ... The experience was fascinating and until the last day it was a joy to revisit a country I had seen briefly as a young naval surgeon. On the last evening I was hit by a speeding stolen car as it mounted a pavement to avoid pursuit. I knew nothing of the episode till I woke in the very same hospital where I had been an external examiner with my leg encased in plaster and the third unit of blood running into my cephalic vein.

Lying there I speculated on what I had heard about the safety of blood in Africa, but by then the Human Immune Virus was busy making acquaintance with my T-lymphocytes..."

F M Hull (from reference 1 below)

The "modern day plague", "the new syphilis", and "the disease from outer space", were all descriptions initially applied to the acquired immunodeficiency syndrome, AIDS. With the discovery of the human immunodeficiency virus (HIV), we became aware of the true nature of the beast, and when the burgeoning epidemic itself became apparent about 1985, medical and scientific resources were mobilised all over the world and a vast amount of information accumulated about it and the virus in a remarkably short time. The biochemical input has been considerable, and although AIDS remains uncurable, has contributed much to the therapeutic possibilities.

AZT AS A BIOCHEMICAL BLOCKER

HIV, in common with other retroviruses, contains the enzyme reverse transcriptase, important for the spread of the virus to other host cells as it enables the viral RNA to be copied to a complementary DNA strand. This in turn can be integrated into the DNA of the host cell, and in turn able to form a new virus by coding for viral proteins.

Even in the face of this knowledge about the viral life cycle, treatment for HIV-1 infection has until recently been somewhat dismal, being only "symptomatic", or "palliative", in other words, unable to get at the root or cause of the condition. Now the first drug licensed for the serious manifestions of HIV-1 infection is available, under the commercial names Zidovudine or Retrovir. It is an analogue of the nucleoside deoxythymidine, 3'-azido-2',3'-dideoxythymidine to be precise, and AZT is a more convenient way to refer to it. Its mode of action is by competition with naturally occurring thymidine by becoming incorporated into the viral DNA chain. Further elongation of the DNA chain is prevented by the azido group of AZT. Once within the cell, AZT becomes phosphorylated and its triphosphate form has at least a one hundred times greater affinity for viral reverse transcriptase than for the host's DNA polymerase.

AZT is generally prescribed when there are serious manifestations of the immunodeficiency of AIDS, such as Kaposi's sarcoma, neurogenic dysfunction like peripheral neuropathy, as well as thrombocytopenia or psoriasis. It has also been suggested that AZT may have an emergency role in combating the great potential tragedy of the AIDS scenario, notably infection of medical personnel due to needlestick injuries or surgeons due to sewing needles and knives (self-injury is reported to occur in 15–20% of surgical operations.) Although even in those circumstances the likelihood of becoming seropositive for HIV is small, nobody wants to contribute to the risk statistics. Further work is needed before AZT can be routinely offered to such victims in the hope of preventing seroconversion.

These are as yet still early days in the optimisation of AZT treatment protocols, although it is worth remembering that because AZT only acts while the genomic DNA is being replicated, it must presumably be given over the long-term and continuously, to interfere with the viral reverse transcriptase before the host's DNA can be invaded. The drug itself has side-effects, some of which can be lethal, such as bone marrow toxicity necessitating repeated transfusions and blood counts.

The search for alternative reverse transcriptase inhibitors continues. Other analogues have been used such as 2,3-dideoxycytidine (DDC) and 2,3-dideoxyinosine (DDI). Warm from the medical press is another group of agents, derived from tetrahydro-imidazol-benzodiazepin-one (TIBO), which appear to have very potent abilities in inhibiting HIV-1 replication, in vitro, with good specificity.

No Entry

Another mode of treatment of HIV infection is to prevent or minimise the entry of the virus into the host cell. The CD4 molecule, an antigen expressed by subsets of human mature T-cells and macrophages, is the receptor for HIV and is known to play a role in T-cell activation, possibly by interacting with major histocompatibility complex class II molecules on the antigen-presenting cells which are involved in the presentation of foreign antigens to T-cell receptors. The envelope glycoprotein gp120 of the virus has a very high binding affinity for the CD4 surface antigen.

There are about 80 molecules of it per virion, and it is highly glycosylated with an unusual structure of loops giving a characteristic knob and spike texture. An important point is that unlike DNA polymerase, reverse transcriptase has a much greater error rate in coding and this results in more rearrangements, point mutations and recombinations in retroviruses than in other viruses. Consequently, AIDS virus glycoproteins have hypervariable regions. This has considerable implications in strategies to design vaccines against the virus — it would be easier to design biologicals as vaccines with a fixed antigenic structure to work from.

gp120 is therefore important for the attachment and entry of HIV into the host cell. Furthermore, CD4 positive cells with bound gp120 can be susceptible to destruction mediated by antibody-dependent cellular cytotoxicity or cytotoxic T-cells of the host. The culmination of these events, i.e. destruction of T-helper cells, interruption of cellular recognition and viral spread to other host cells, contributes to the immunopathology of HIV infection.

Significant too is the work on the protease cleavage of gp120, which incorporates an area, designated as the V3 loop, particularly rich in arginine and alanine residues, and a major site for eliciting neutralising antibodies. If this V3 region is cleaved by certain proteases, then these neutralising antibodies are unable to recognise gp120, although in the cleaved state it is still able to bind to CD4. It is possible therefore that a specific cleavage of gp120 at the V3 loop is necessary for viral infection. This suggests a therapeutic attack on the virus, in the form of a protease inhibitor of some sort, as the cleavage may result in conformational changes of the gp120 molecule, facilitating its binding to the CD4 molecule and the uptake of the virus into the host's cell, otherwise blocked by the host's neutralising antibodies.

DECOYS

Another therapeutic possibility is to use soluble CD4 as a so-called "decoy" molecule to mop up HIV particles or unbound gp120 molecules before they can bind to host cells. A form of soluble CD4 that expresses the gp120 binding domain area is available from gene insertion into cultured cells. It has to be given intramuscularly or intravenously but has been used in initial clinical trials in HIV infection. The fear, of course, is that this in itself could lead to an immune response in the host, as the CD4 molecule is fundamental to the whole immune system. This fear seems, if not groundless, to be mitigated by the fact that although the N-terminal end of the CD4 molecule is responsible for both interaction with major histocompatibility complex class II molecules of antigen presenting cells and also gp120 binding, the precise regions involved in these events are different. One related option is the possibility of raising an antibody directed against the gp120 binding site of the CD4 molecule, i.e an anti-idiotype, that is to say an antibody directed against the antigen combining site of another antibody.

One can see that the possibilities, based upon a knowledge of the structural and functional characteristics of the cell's response to the virus infection, are many and varied. Human ingenuity and viral persistence/adaptation are in direct conflict here; the consensus appears to be that, in the end, the virus has no chance.

METABOLIC CRISIS IN AIDS

Most clinical effort has devolved on the fatal complications of opportunistic infections due to the immunodeficiency in AIDS patients, but sufferers also experience a progressive and unexplained weight loss. It is not the usual type of starvation, wherein mostly fat is removed; in AIDS there is a selective disappearance of lean body mass, mostly muscle. Remarkably, it has been pointed out that in AIDS, sufficient lean body mass may be lost for that to be a cause of death in itself. Since potassium is largely an intracellular cation, this wasting of lean mass can be followed by measuring total body potassium, and typically the largest amounts are lost in the nine or so months before death. In terms of weight *per se*, the loss is usually about 34% before death. Kotler even managed to produce an apposite, but chilling formula:

$$\text{days from death} = \frac{54 - \% \text{ K}}{0.17}$$

where % K is the total body potassium as a percentage of normal. It is easily calculated that when potassium reaches about half of what is normal then there is not long to go. (In the way that the formula is arranged, the result comes out negative, which however seems appropriate.) What is the cause of this circumstance, unexpectedly almost as dire as the immune dysfunction? Paradoxically, it is probably a defect in lipid metabolism. Normal weight loss would involve a regulated and economic use of stored fat for energy purposes when there is anorexia, malabsorption, or the hypermetabolism of infection. In AIDS this does not take place and a dangerous alternative, the mobilisation of protein stores from lean tissue, takes its place.

The pathophysiological reasons for weight loss in AIDS are speculative, but are likely to be multiple. Certainly food intake may be inadequate due to loss of appetite and infections of the gastrointestinal tract, e.g. oesophagitis caused by the fungus *Candida albicans*. The gastrointestinal tract may also be implicated due to the malabsorption syndromes common in AIDS patients. Anorexia may also be a side-effect of medication. There is also evidence that tumour necrosis factor, otherwise known as cachectin (since it is thought to cause the cachexia of cancer) may also be involved. It is primarily a macrophage, not a T-cell product, in response to infection (Chap. 17b). Yet again, it seems that unlike in most debilitating illnesses, triiodothyronine secretion is unimpaired in AIDS, and this would lead to weight loss in the face of chronic illness and malnutrition.

Here is yet another field in which we await answers, and beyond that, some remedial strategy. Meanwhile, we might recall that in central Africa AIDS is known as the "slim disease".

ENVOI

An elementary knowledge of nucleic acid and protein biochemistry can materially help one's understanding of the immunology and the therapeutic approach to AIDS, allowing an appreciation of advances as they come off the press, and they come rapidly. Apart from the weighty pieces involving epidemiology and therapeutics, there are certain fascinating tidbits. The earliest known case of a definite HIV positive serum has, until recently, been considered to be one taken in Zaire in 1959. Early in 1990 though, workers in Manchester extracted DNA from the paraffin sections relating to the case of a sailor who had died in 1959 of cytomegalovirus and pneumocystic infection. Sure enough, the DNA contained HIV sequences. Why did the disease not spread in Manchester at that time? The wife of the seaman and the youngest of the three daughters, presumably infected by him, died soon after him, and with similar symptomology. As the journal *Nature* put it, an isolated infection like this may run into the sand, a personal tragedy only. But now we know that at least two adults died of AIDS in 1959. Why did it suddenly spread in the late 1970s? There have been many attempts at an explanation, but consider an interesting one — because, since the 1960s people's dietary, but not their sexual habits, changed markedly, is AIDS in essence a nutritional disease?

Further Reading

1. Hull FM. If I were HIV positive. *Br J of Clin Pract.* **42** : 357–358, 1988 (A fictional scenario).
2. Anonymous. What do we know about the mechanism of weight loss in AIDS. *Nutrition Reviews* **48** : 153–154, 1990.
3. Schild GC and Minor PD. Human immunodeficiency virus and AIDS: challenges and progress. *Lancet* **335** : 1081–1084, 1990.
4. Corbitt G, Bailey AS and Williams G. HIV infection in Manchester, 1959. *Lancet* **336** : 51, 1990. (See also "Comment" in *Nature* **346** : 92, 1990.

3c

Cystic Fibrosis:
Working the New Gene

"The biggest problem of modern genetics is one we have scarcely come to terms with: the ubiquity of genetic disease."
— Steve Jones (in the Reith Lectures, 1991)

Cystic fibrosis (CF), originally called cystic disease of the pancreas (the more descriptive name **mucoviscidosis** did not catch on) is well known as one of these diseases which has a markedly ethnic distribution; it occurs in 1 in 2000 live births in Caucasians, less frequently (1 : 17 000) in blacks, but is very rare in Asians. It is characterised by an unduly thick and viscous secretion from all the exocrine glands. Remarkably, it is in a sense a "new" disease, for it only became well known in the antibiotic era. Previously, children whose lungs and pancreas produced the sticky mucous came down with pneumonia and malabsorption and these were regarded as the real cause of death. Now survival is much prolonged by penicillin and other antibiotics (with a big improvement evident on introducing aminoglycosides into the small airways by aerosols) on the one hand, and the oral administration of pancreatic enzymes on the other. Patients are also helped by special physiotherapy techniques. Survival (now usually into the mid-twenties) has promoted recognition and investigation of the primary disease.

The traditional means of diagnosis has been by analysis of serum trypsin (related to dysfunction of the exocrine pancreas; as the disease progresses immunoreactive trypsin declines) or sodium and/or chloride in sweat. In CF the defect in epithelial transport leads to a sweat with a high salt content; the parasympathomimetic drug pilocarpine is injected into the skin and the resulting secretion collected on a piece of weighed filter paper or in a capillary tube for the analysis. These methods are evidently only applicable after birth, and even there there are problems, for sweat is often collected from babies with much difficulty. The aim has been to devise:

(1) Effective detection of carriers to allow genetic counselling.
(2) Early prenatal detection (there have been tests for prenatal detection based upon alkaline phosphatase isoenzymes in the amniotic fluid, but they have

turned out to very difficult to put into practice).

(3) Beyond these, some specific therapy for the defect itself rather than its concequences.

THE NEW GENE

If there is a history of CF in the family, then couples are of course alerted, but due to the high carrier frequency (some 1 in 25 of any population of European descent is a heteozygote) most infants with disease are born into families which cannot identify any previously known victims. Screening therefore has to be applied to couples before pregnancy or early in pregnancy, with subsequent prenatal diagnosis and termination if desired. Such a programme might seem unexceptionable, but screening an adult population for heterozygosity in relation to a genetic defect is not a common procedure. It has been done successfully, nonetheless, for thalassaemia in Cyprus and for Tay-Sachs disease in Ashkenazi Jews. And it is precisely because CF is such a serious disease that there is opposition to screening for it; that is, it is held that there is no good reason for the early detection of a disease for which there is no cure. Moreover, it is feared that in general population screening programmes there might be stigmatisation of heterozygotes. However, on the other side of the argument there are well over 2 million heterozygotes in UK alone, a lot of people to try to stigmatise if you are that way inclined, and in extension, it has to be emphasised by public education that we all carry deleterious mutations of one sort or another. The most cogent argument for screening, of course, is that it gives choice — to prospective parents, to pregnant women, and not least, to doctors in respect of an early choice of therapy.

Nonetheless, if you want to screen effectively, the programme must elicit very few false positives and negatives, and this has hitherto been the problem with such biochemical tests as were possible for CF in the foetus. Moreover, there was no test for the carrier state in adults. It was realised a few years ago that the new genetics might offer a way round these difficulties if only the gene could be located and its mutations probed with a complementary DNA. The situation is that, if in investigating a disease, you know there is production of an abnormal protein, you can (nowadays) sequence that protein, either in the normal or abnormal form, synthesise a DNA probe corresponding to all or part of that amino acid sequence, and use it to locate the region on the chromosome, or on a fragment of the full genomic DNA, after restriction endonuclease digestion. (Such is the case for sickle cell anaemia, for example.) However, for CF the nature of any abnormal protein produced was unknown, and it has still not been definitively located. But the investigating scientists were not stumped. They managed to localise the gene to chromosome 7 by studying families affected. They then looked for a known gene near the CF gene. The idea of this is that proximity will make sure the two stay together during recombination (the shuffling of genetic material during meoisis) and that any substitution in the CF gene will alter the total pattern of DNA fragments from that particular region during restriction endonuclease digestion (Fig. 13). A marker gene called IRP (for *int*-related protein, *int* being an oncogene) was located. The approach did yield a probe which was informative in many families, although usually there has to have been an affected individual for comparison.

In 1989, Tsui and Collins announced that they had found the CF gene itself. This was done by detecting markers on either side of the CF gene (the new ones were the *met* oncogene and a sequence known as T3.11) and finding the frequency with which they were passed down from parent to child in affected families (again on the principle that the nearer they are on the chromosome, the less likely they are to become detached during meiosis). By continually breaking the DNA up and comparing sequence after sequence, they worked their way along the chromosome, finding expressed regions which corresponded to sequences from other animals, that is, conserved sequences coding for functional proteins. Eventually they found one which corresponded to the mRNA of a cloned sequence from sweat glands, which is one of the main tissues in which the CF gene is expressed (hence the high sweat chloride). The gene itself turned out to be quite large, 250 kilobases, with no less than 24 exons, separated by non-coding introns. With probes for the whole gene, there will be no need for tracking family members, and screening can be conducted on adults for carrier status, or on foetuses, or newborns as desired. The laboratory will only require as starting material some cells with a little intact DNA, leucocytes remaining the most popular for the time being. However, it is likely that hair roots or cheek scrapings will become routine in the next few years. The sequence of operations is outlined in Fig. 12.

THE DEFECT

Here is a disease then, in which the precise defect was unknown before characterisation of the gene, but the base sequence of the gene allowed prediction of the amino acid sequence of the protein expressed, plus a guess at its three-dimensional structure. It turns out to have the hydrophobic domains typical of a transmembrane protein, consistent with the long-standing theory that it constitutes a chloride channel, and it has been called the cystic fibrosis transmembrane conductance regulator (CFTR). Now synthesised and cloned, it turns out that it requires phosphorylation and energy input (ATP hydrolysis) before it opens. Deletion of a single phenylalanine residue at position 508 (the deltaF508 mutation) is the most common mutation leading to the disease. This makes detection by the polymerase chain reaction (see preceeding chapter) quite feasible for prenatal and carrier detection. It does not help if the mutation is unknown, when the techniques using restriction endonucleases, as described above, will still be required.

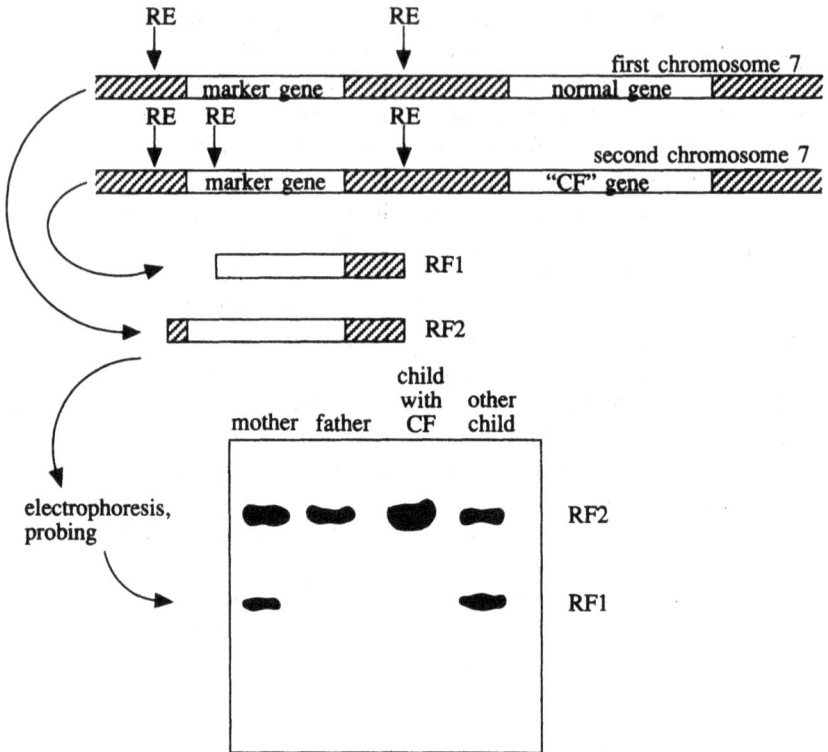

Fig. 13 Use of linkage analysis to detect a cystic fibrosis carrier.

In this illustration there is a nuclear family of two parents, and two children, one of whom has CF. It is highly desirable to know whether the unaffected child is a carrier. (Of course both parents must be carriers for this autosomal recessive condition.) The gene for CF not being located at the time this method was developed, a gene known to be near to the CF gene (and to have polymorphisms susceptible to detection by restriction endonucleases) is selected and complementary DNA probes prepared for it. After digestion of the genomic DNA with restriction endonuclease these probes are used to detect the restriction fragments separated by electrophoresis. Here the mother, yielding two bands, appears to be heterozygous for the marker alleles, whereas the father is homozygous, giving one band only, and so is considered to be uninformative. But since the affected child inherited the allele RF2 from both parents, it would appear to be associated with the disease, and RF1 is probably associated with the normal gene. Thus the preliminary indications are that this child is not a carrier; the chances can be computed on a knowledge of the inheritance pattern of the marker locus used. In practice, other restriction enzymes catalysing scission at other polymorphic sites will be used to try to make the father informative and to narrow down the chances one way or the other.

RE = restriction endonuclease
RF = restriction fragment

Anyway, we are finding out now why children with the disease, even before it was scientifically characterised, were remarkable for their "salty skin" and we shall soon be reading reports of clinical trials of CFTR introduced directly into the lungs.

Further Reading

1. Dodge JA. Implications of the new genetics for screening for cystic fibrosis. *Lancet* **2** : 672–673,1988.
2. Ringe D and Petsko GA. Cystic fibrosis: a transport problem. *Nature* **346** : 312–313, 1990.
3. Marx JL. The cystic fibrosis gene is found. *Science* **245** : 923–925, 1989.
4. Wine JJ. The mutant protein responds. *Nature* **354** : 503–504, 1991.

3d

Cell Energy Supply — Crisis? — What Crisis?

Every cell in the body needs a constant supply of at least two substances — oxygen and glucose. The latter may be substituted from time to time by alternatives such as amino acids, fatty acids, ketones and other sugars, but in general these are adaptations in the face of some metabolic stress. Some tissues, notably the brain, are however dependent upon having at least a modicum of glucose for normal functioning — other fuels may replace it only to a limited extent. There is no substitute for oxygen, however, in any organ or tissue.

Energy deficit in the brain due to glucose and/or oxygen starvation is easily detected (in instances where external injury or infection can be excluded) in that the subject becomes confused or unconscious (disordered sensorium). With other tissues, the task may not be so easy. But what diseases/stresses cause cell energy crisis, and what cells are at risk? To show the extensive spread of this branch of metabolic medicine, we can list them as follows:

(1) Intense physical stress
(2) Starvation
(3) Glycogen storage disease
(4) Fructose intolerance
(5) Alcoholic intoxication
(6) Adult repiratory distress syndrome
(7) Burns
(8) Haemorrhagic and other types of shock (including heart attacks).

This seems an ill-assorted list, but all of them are associated with a dramatic rise, in the blood, of a substance easily and quickly measured in hospital laboratories, namely uric acid. Revision of some basic biochemistry will reveal why this is so and why monitoring uric acid concentrations will lead to better understanding of the condition of the patient. Of course prolonged hyperuricaemia is often associated with a primary increase in uric acid production and is manifested as gout. Here we are discussing a range of alternative reasons.

PURINE CATABOLISM

Every cell of course needs a constant supply of ATP, whose synthesis and consumption are well balanced in the normal unstressed cell. Synthesis is regulated above all by oxygen and glucose availability but when these are lacking there is net consumption to meet essential metabolic requirements and ATP degradation products, intially ADP and AMP, accumulate. Their futher catabolism, enhanced when there is compromised resynthesis, is reviewed in Fig. 14. In humans, the end product is uric acid which is therefore a prime marker for energy crisis. It is however, evidently a "sink" for all the purine metabolites, some of which might potentially be better indices, the more so as they sometimes have biological effects in themselves .

Adenosine, especially, is a powerful effector and causes, *inter alia,* vasodilation. It has been proposed as a beneficial agent in cardioplegic arrest. It also has a suppressive effect on neutrophil activity, potentially applicable to hyperimmune conditions such as asthma. Xanthine and hypoxanthine are also of interest. When the enzyme xanthine oxidase is called on to remove surges of xanthine, it forms free radicals, that is highly reactive and damaging fragments of whole molecules. The significance of this is still not entirely clear.

Probably practising clinicians will soon be able to send blood to the laboratory for xanthine and/or adenosine assays, and will be able to interpret them along the lines suggested for uric acid below, but with more precision.

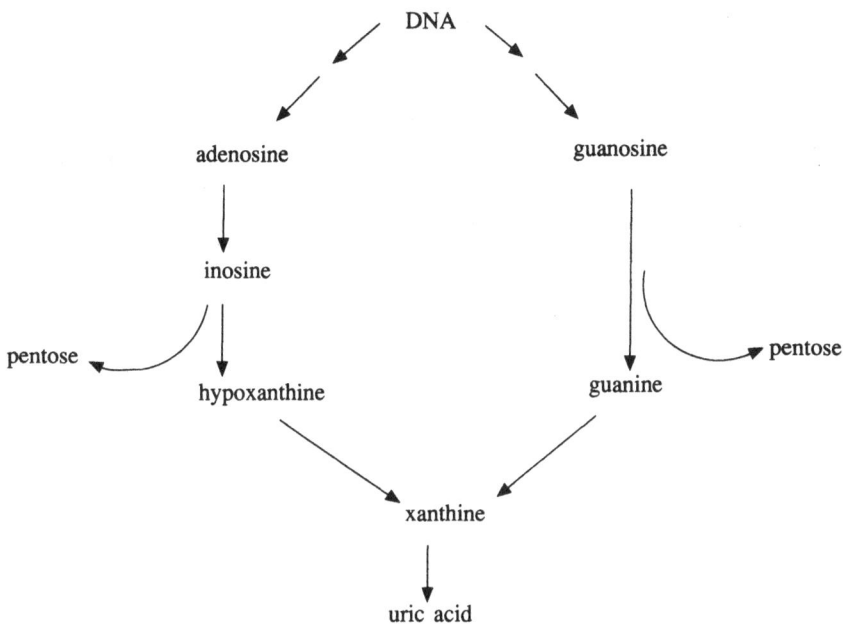

Fig. 14   A reminder of the main steps in purine catabolism.

ALCOHOLIC INTOXICATION

Alcohol produces what is thought to be a hypermetabolic state, that is the turnover of substrates is enhanced without necessarily any concomitant increase in glucose and/or oxygen to support it. So ATP is used up without complete replenishment. Hyperuricaemia occurs in fasting alcoholics for another reason. In the fasting state blood glucose has to be maintained from amino acids by gluconeogenesis. But this pathway is routed through pyruvate. When alcohol is ingested in the fasting state there is an oversufficiency of reduced nucleotide, NADH, and the pyruvate tends to be trapped as lactate. Not only can this lead to hypoglycaemia, but the lactate competes with urate for excretion by the tubules of the kidney.

In addition, after an acute dose of alcohol, there is a surge of acetate; for disposal of this as acetyl CoA, ATP is used up, and this contributes further to the nucleotide breakdown. The three mechanisms cited as producing hyperuricaemia are then:

(1) relative energy lack in relation to metabolic activity
(2) lactic acidosis
(3) acetate disposal

GLYCOGEN STORAGE DISEASE

There are of course some eight types of glycogen storage disease well dealt with in basic biochemistry since they illustrate the importance of the carbohydrate economy in the liver. The defects become apparent in early childhood, but because different enzymes and different tissues are involved, the clinical course is variable. In general there is a failure of glucose homeostasis, since after all the store of liver glycogen serves to buffer fluctuations in blood glucose. The most common of the variants is deficiency of glucose 6-phosphatase, Type I or von Gierke's disease (of which a case is related in Chap. 7a). In this situation, glucose entering the liver from the portal system undergoes rapid phosphorylation with consequent ATP depletion, and any glycogen synthesised is unavailable as a source of glucose as there is little or no enzyme to hydrolyse glucose phosphates to glucose for release into the systemic circulation. There is a characteristic picture of hypoglycaemia, hyperlipidaemia, lactic acidosis, and hyperuricaemia. To combat the first of these, some patients have been given glucose infusions via an indwelling catheter served by a pump of the type used to titrate diabetics with insulin — the so-called artificial pancreas, although in this context it is more of an artificial liver, designed conversely to raise the levels of blood glucose. Under such circumstances, the efficacy of the treatment can be assessed by measuring lactic acid, triglycerides, or uric acid in the blood — it is of little use trying to interpret blood glucose concentrations to assess the patient's status if you are engaged in administering glucose itself. Of the three candidates, uric acid is probably the easiest and cheapest to analyse.

FRUCTOSE INTOLERANCE

Children who react badly to fructose (usually in the form of sucrose) may be lacking any one of the enzymes necessary to metabolise it. If a lack of fructokinase is the culprit, then there is no uricaemia since ATP cannot be used up. In the case of the other two, the transferase and the epimerase (cf. Fig. 8) the dose of fructose is rapidly taken up by the liver in a noninsulin-dependent manner and phosphorylated by ATP which cannot be replenished as further metabolism of the fructose phosphate is blocked. Thus there is hyperuricaemia. Fortunately, we can survive without fructose, which must merely be eliminated from the diet.

RESPIRATORY DISTRESS SYNDROME

Adult respiratory distress syndrome is a multivalent condition associated with hypoxic energy crisis arising in tissues and cells outside the lung. It is a "new" disease (circa 1967) which is still much argued over, but was so named because lung biopsies suggested a similarity to infantile respiratory distress syndrome. Some deleterious mechanism leads to pulmonary oedema and reduced total lung capacity. However, it is fatal in over 50% of established cases and a rapid rise in serum uric acid should be a warning signal of increasing danger.

HYPERURICAEMIA AS A GRAVE PROGNOSTIC SIGN

Finally, consider starvation and debilitating exercise/hard labour. They are evidently akin to each other, in that there is energy demand with glucose available neither from food nor from bodily stores to supply it. In severe exercise, in addition, there is a degree of muscle destruction accompanied by tearing and haemorrhagic lesions. It is rare for athletes to fall ill and die whilst running except from heart attacks, but energy crisis deaths were predicted for the Mexico City Olympic games some years ago, on the predication of extra hypoxic stress at high altitude. If a person ill from inanation, hard labour, dehydration, or burns shows a steadily rising uric acid in spite of aggressive therapy, then the prognosis is grave.

Further Reading

1. Fox IH, Palella TD and Kelley WN. Hyperuricaemia: a marker for cell energy crisis. *New Engl. J Med* **317** : 111–112, 1987.
2. Fox IH. Adenosine triphosphate degradation in specific disease. *J Lab Clin Med* **106** : 101–110, 1985.

4a

A Type of Gift Wrapping

We need to move fat around our blood vessels, for it provides energy (triglycerides) and structural components (cholesterol and phospholipids), but this is done at some peril to ourselves. Fat has to be dispersed as comparatively small particles, namely the lipoproteins, in which the protein acts as a sort of packaging, stabilising the droplets in the aqueous environment of the plasma. If fat is allowed to coalesce into large clumps it causes occlusion and hypoxia, for example in the fat embolism after a crushing injury to bone. Added to that, free fatty acids are toxic, mainly by virtue of their haemolytic effect, and for transport they form their own innocuous protein complex, with albumin.

If the lipoprotein particles are to deliver fats to cells for energy and structural integrity they have to be recognised, and it is the function of receptors on the cell membrane to do this. It was the physiologists who first described receptors, in respect of hormones like adrenaline and also the acetylcholine receptors in synapses, so that lipoprotein receptors were rather late on the scene; however, due to their enormous public health importance in relation to heart disease, we now know a great deal about them. They are an essential component of the integrated transport of lipid, which however, is not so integrated that it can easily be explained or summarised. Nonetheless, one can at least separately consider the fates of exogenous and endogenous lipid.

Exogenous or dietary lipid becomes incorporated into chylomicron particles in the small intestinal mucosa, which also synthesises apolipoprotein B48 for incorporation into them. Under the action of the enzyme lipoprotein lipase, in the endothelia of the capillary beds of muscle and adipose tissue, the chylomicron triglyceride is split and they become "remnants" which are taken up by the liver. These liver receptors recognise apolipoprotein E, acquired from other lipoproteins in the circulation. The fatty acids released during the production of remnants are taken up by the tissues (Fig. 15). This whole process would not occur were not apolipoprotein CII also picked up by chylomicrons from other lipoproteins in the circulation, for CII is an activator of lipoprotein lipase. Another such activator is insulin; this is only to be expected, since insulin release and activity is always a response to feeding, serving to incorporate substrates into cells.

The endogenous lipoprotein pathway begins with the synthesis by the liver of very low density lipoproteins (VLDL) which are principally triglyceride, though they have some cholesterol and cholesterol ester, and have as their main "apo" an extended version of B48, called B100. VLDL triglycerides are also hydrolysed by CII-activated lipoprotein lipase during their passage through the capillary beds, so they become progressively smaller and cholesterol enriched, eventually forming the intermediate density lipoproteins (IDLs) which in turn can either be taken up by receptors in the liver or converted to low density lipoproteins (LDLs) (Fig. 16). LDL is the major transporter of cholesterol and cholesterol ester to the tissues and its only apolipoprotein is B100.

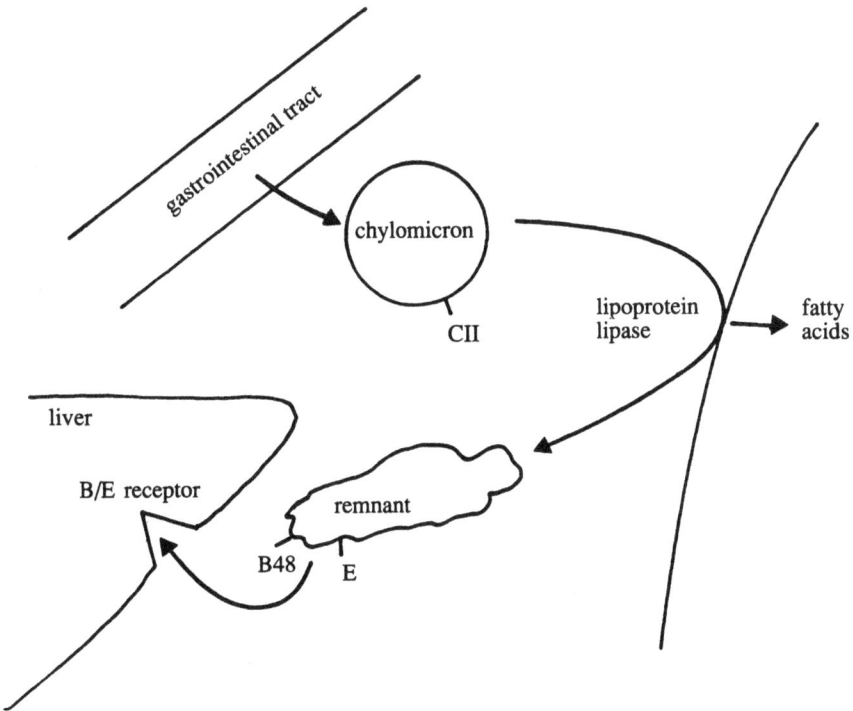

Fig. 15   Assimilation of dietary triglycerides.

The chylomicrons reach the blood via the lymphatics, and are discharged by means of their apolipoprotein CII component activating lipoprotein lipase. The remnants are taken up by the liver.

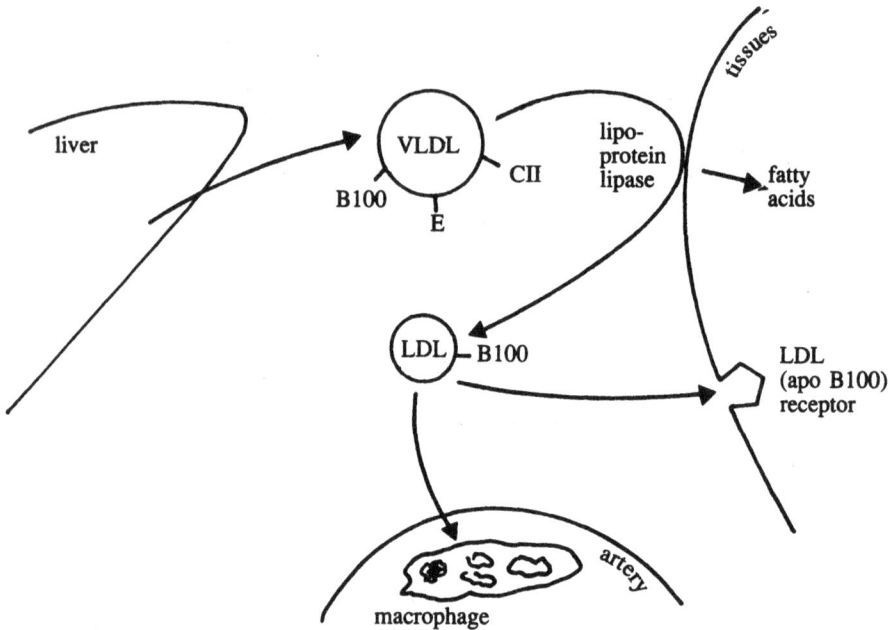

Fig. 16   Mechanisms of transport of endogenous lipids.

VLDL containing triglyceride and cholesterol yields the cholesterol and apolipoprotein B100-rich LDL particle after discharge of the fatty acids at the endothelium of the capillary beds of the muscles and adipose tissue. Cholesterol is supplied to cells by receptor-mediated endocytosis of LDL but there is an alternative uptake system by macrophages. When such macrophages are in the arterial intima they may contribute as foam cells to the atherosclerotic lesion.

Receptor-Mediated Endocytosis

The LDL receptor is expressed by many cells, notably in the liver, and recognises apo B100. In addition, it has also a high affinity for apo E, which helps to explain the binding of IDL particles (which are rich in it). Having bound to the receptor the LDL particles are taken up by the cell by adsorptive endocytosis, followed by endocytic vesicle formation and fusion with lysosomes. Its B100 is hydrolysed to amino acids by lysosomal proteases, its cholesterol esters by lysosomal acid lipase to free cholesterol, which then crosses the lysosomal membrane to the cytoplasm.

The internalised LDL receptor meanwhile can recycle back to the cell surface, to the so-called "coated pit." When the cholesterol requirements of the cell are diminished there is reduction in the expression of surface LDL receptors by a negative feedback control, so inhibiting further cholesterol uptake. So the LDL receptor is essential both for locking the LDL on to the recipient cell and also for regulating the amount of cholesterol taken up by it.

FAMILIAL HYPERCHOLESTEROLAEMIA

What makes the LDL receptor so important clinically is its reduced expression in familial hypercholesterolaemia (FH), a genetic disease inherited in an autosomal recessive manner. Sufferers have high blood cholesterol values and often present with severe atherosclerosis, perhaps in the third decade of life if heterozygous, but even under ten years if homozygous. Prominent stigmata of the disease are the xanthomas, due to macrophages laden with cholesterol causing nodular swellings along the tendons, particularly of the knees and elbows, and also the Achilles tendons as well as the extensor tendons in the hands. The macrophages also have LDL receptors and represent a secondary mechanism for the removal of it from the plasma, evidently an emergency measure (there is evidence that they may serve to scavenge damaged LDL) and not without its disadvantages. Apart from in the xanthomas, cholesterol-laden macrophages (foam cells) are found in the fatty streaks and atheromas destined to form a locus for thrombosis and ischaemia.

The gene for the somatic, physiological LDL receptor is located on the short arm of chromosome 19 and codes for a protein consisting of 839 amino acids. Carbohydrate is linked to this protein in the Golgi bodies, with the production of the mature glycoprotein receptor. It has been structurally divided into five main domains with diverse functions, only one of which is the IDL/LDL binding region recognising apos B100 and E. This segment also has homology with complement C9 and the clotting protein thrombomodulin, suggesting that in modified form it might have something to do with thrombosis. The middle portion consists of a large span that is in part homologous with the epidermal growth factor precursor. A membrane spanning domain anchors the LDL receptor to the cell surface membrane, while the carboxyl terminal end consists of a cytoplasmic domain involved in the localisation of the receptor in the coated pit regions of the cell membrane.

With such a complex molecular entity, there is obviously the potential for numerous structural variants, and Goldstein and Brown have described four main classes of mutation, resulting in different variants of FH:

Class 1 mutations — failure of LDL receptor synthesis.

Class 2 mutations — the receptor is synthesised but is incorrectly transported to the cell membrane for expression, probably due to some defect in the Golgi apparatus.

Class 3 mutations — a defect in the ligand binding domain, so that affinity is poor or non-existent.

Class 4 mutations — the receptor is either lost from the cell membrane, implying a disorder of the membrane-spanning domain, or there is a defect in the internalisation process.

As a consequence of any of these, there is decreased clearance from the serum of LDL (and IDL, which shares the receptor).

REVERSE CHOLESTEROL TRANSPORT, LECITHIN AND THE HEALTH FOOD SHOPS

Since most (if by no means all) substances in the blood and the body are held in some sort of homeostatic balance, there is a mechanism for *removing* cholesterol from cell surfaces as well as for depositing it there. This is often termed reverse cholesterol transport, and involves high density lipoprotein (HDL) particles, richer in protein and phospholipid than VLDL and LDL. HDL is synthesisied in the liver and probably donates apo CII to the chylomicrons and apo E to both chylomicrons and VLDL remnants as it encounters them in the serum. They also contribute phospholipid substrate for the lecithin cholesterol acyl transferase (LCAT) reaction which esterifies the cholesterol on cell surfaces. This reaction requires apo AI as activator. The cholesterol ester is incorporated into the nascent HDL, which gradually becomes more spheroid, and is finally taken up by the liver via receptors still poorly characterised (Fig. 17). The whole pathway can be regarded as excretory, for in the liver the cholesterol is partially converted to bile salts, which despite the enterohepatic circulation eventually end up being eliminated in the faeces. The body can synthesise the steroid nucleus with ease but has no means to break it up, only to modify it for excretion in the bile.

The fact that an essential component of the cholesterol excretory pathway is lecithin, properly known as phosphatidyl choline, and commercially extracted from egg yolk and soya beans, did not escape the notice of the health food industry, and it has been much advertised as a substance capable of cleaning up your arteries. Choline itself has had the status of a quasi-vitamin for some decades; nevertheless, its essentialness has never been demonstrated for humans, albeit that it prevents fatty liver in rats. No trial has yet been able to show that lecithin is hypocholesterolaemic in a human population; it is just possible that it is hypocholesterolaemic in some idiosyncratic subjects — the problem is, how to find them?

The metabolic and epidemiological indications then are that HDL should be as high as possible, and total and LDL cholesterol should be low, but there is still room for much interpretation.

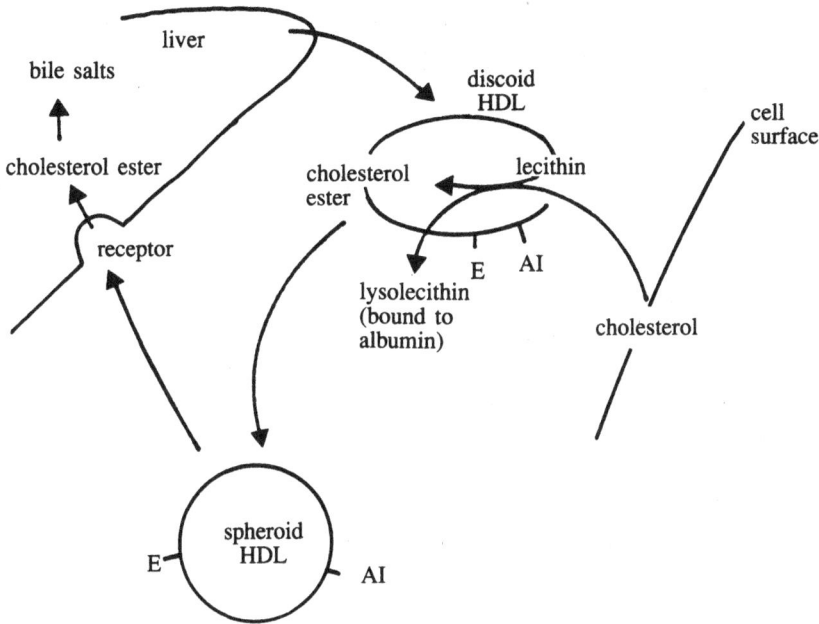

Fig. 17 Concept of reverse cholesterol transport.

Discoid HDL, assembled in the liver, is able to remove cholesterol from cell membranes by esterifying it with an acyl group from phospholipid, catalysed by lecithin cholesterol acyl transferase. Apolipoprotein AI is necessary for the activation of the enzyme. The cholesterol ester is incorporated into the HDL particle which acquires a more spheroid shape and is taken up by the liver in a process probably dependent on the recognition of apolipoprotein E by a receptor. In the liver there is a mechanism of excretion for the steroid nucleus via conversion to bile salts.

PATIENTS AND PRUDENCE

The lipid clinic at a hospital screened a 50-year-old man with no specific complaints and the laboratory found the following:

total	cholesterol	7.54 mmol/l
HDL	cholesterol	2.32 mmol/l
LDL	cholesterol	4.20 mmol/l
VLDL	cholesterol	0.25 mmol/l
triglycerides		0.75 mmol/l

The consultant noted that the total cholesterol was quite high, above the 90th percentile for his age and sex. This would call for vigorous intervention were it not partly attributable to a rather high HDL cholesterol, which was above the 95th percentile for the same age and sex. There would not then seem to be anything to worry about. However, the consultant noticed that there is a missing quantum of cholesterol somewhere within the results above. The subfractions of cholesterol (HDL + LDL + VLDL) do not add up to the total, leaving a gap of 0.77 mmol/l. Since triglycerides and VLDL (its main carrier) are both low, they are internally consistent, and it seems likely that either HDL or LDL cholesterol is reported as lower than the correct concentration. It is hoped that this inconsistency will be sorted out when the lipid profile is repeated in a few months, but in the meantime, since total cholesterol is undoubtedly high, and LDL cholesterol *may* be higher than it seems, the consultant thought it best to advise the adoption of a prudent diet — cutting down drastically on dairy products, organ and fatty meats, and the consumption of moderate amounts of fibre.

The case illustrates some of the uncertainties which may arise — what to do if both total and HDL cholesterol are high and how to cope with apparent lack of accuracy in laboratory measurements. Holding a watching brief and giving some dietary advice seemed the most sensible course.

CHOLESTEROL AND CANCER

Your patients will be able, perhaps eager, to read the health columns of newspapers and magazines and will not hestitate to ask you whether, in persuading them to try to lower their serum cholesterol with miserable diets and gigantic pills, you are not exposing them to an enhanced risk of cancer. This quite novel *via dolorosa* was uncovered after several clinical trials of hypocholesterolaemic drugs. It was observed that the total (i.e., non-cardiovascular) mortality of the groups which enjoyed a reduction in serum cholesterol showed no improvement over the control (placebo) groups. There was no single cause of death in the former, but the data suggested that both cancer and violent death were prominent. Meta-analysis (a way of combining separate clinical trials in a single statistical treatment) showed that the relation between drug intervention and cancer was probably not causal but there was suspicion of a causal link with violent death. Can serum cholesterol be too low as well as too high?

AN EXTREME CASE OF HYPOCHOLESTEROLAEMIA

Dr Anne Bauer writes (in ref 4 below) that she was consulted by an elderly man complaining of gastrointestinal discomfort and weight loss. This turned out after suitable examination and testing (presence of antinuclear antibodies) to be due to disseminated discoid lupus erythematosus. Despite drug therapy, he failed to improve and at one point a complete chemistry profile was sought. It was unremarkable except for a strikingly low serum cholesterol, at 1.1. mmol/l. At once a thyroid panel was ordered, for serum cholesterol is low in hyperthyroidism; on the contrary, however, the patient turned out to be mildly hypothyroid, if anything. Disseminated lupus erythematosus, an autoimmune disease, often has gastrointestinal symptoms and these were approached by means of metronidazole to eliminate bacterial overgrowth and also the provision of a modified diet containing mainly medium chain triglcyerides, which can be largely hydrolysed in the stomach, as opposed to the small intestine. After one month his condition improved and his serum cholesterol rose to 2.3 mmol/l.

Evidently, the low serum cholesterol has been a signal of the seriousness of his condition. Not only could he not absorb cholesterol, it seemed that he could not synthesise it in his liver either, although standard function tests had indicated the liver to be healthy. A low serum cholesterol may therefore be added to the list of prognostic markers (Chap. 7a); it drops in the terminal stages of the AIDS syndrome, for example, along with total body potassium. Indeed it drops in most viral infections (although not catastrophically) and it is worth asking your patients if they have been suffering from a cold or flu before you proceed to measure it and try to interpret it in the context of the risk of heart disease.

Comment

It is of course most decidedly the received medical opinion that a high blood cholesterol concentration carries a strong, implicitly causal association with coronary heart disease and that aggressive intervention should be instituted to reduce it, at least in pre-middle-aged subjects who might have other risk factors, like a family history of sudden cardiac death. But not all authorities are happy, in particular about what is meant by "high" and whether studies on middle-aged men, the group thought to be most at risk, can be transposed across the board, to women for example. Studies of blood lipids relation to disease in women are only now getting underway. For many years to come, a scrutiny of the quality literature will be very essential to deal with this topic sensibly, to avoid being swayed by zealots, oversimplifiers, and the numerous parties with vested interests.

Further Reading

1. Erkelens DW. Apolipoproteins in lipid transport, an impressionist view. *Postgrad Med J* **65** : 275–281, 1989.
2. Brown MS and Goldstein JL. Scavenging for receptors. *Nature* **343** : 508–509, 1990.

3. Muldoon MF, Manuck SB and Mathews KA. Lowering cholesterol concentrations and mortality: a quantitative review of primary prevention trials. *Br Med J* **301** : 309–3124, 1990.

4. Anon. Severe acquired hypocholesterolaemia: two case reports. *Nutrition Reviews* **47**, 202–207, 1989.

4b

Flip-Flop

Although the title of this section may suggest some sort of acrobatic exercise in a weight watchers' class, the term refers instead to molecular gymnastics involving certain negatively charged phospholipids such as phosphatidylserine within the plasma membrane of platelets. Platelets have the ability to convert prothrombin to thrombin, an activity termed prothrombinase expression. This reaction takes place at the cell surface and involves a complex of coagulation factors Va and Xa, in the presence of calcium ions and a negatively charged phospholipid environment. In addition, platelets are also capable of activating coagulation factor X to form Xa in the presence of IXa and VIIIa, with the formation of the tenase complex, likewise using calcium ions and a suitable negatively charged phospholipid surface (Fig. 18).

The negatively charged phospholipid surface of platelets in these reactions, which incidentally may be expressed by other blood cells, should not be thought of as a static surface, but as a highly dynamic environment, with the capacity to provide a catalytic surface for coagulation events. The negatively charged phospholipids such as phosphatidylserine can bind to particular coagulation factors such as Xa and prothrombin, and markedly increase the efficiency of the reactions in terms of lowered Km (i.e. enhanced substrate binding) and raised maximum velocity.

There are topological considerations for the distribution of negatively charged phospholipids within the plasma membrane. It has been shown that in unactivated platelets, phosphatidylserine lies predominantly at the **inner** leaflet of the lipid membrane bilayer; however, upon platelet activation by such agonists as thrombin

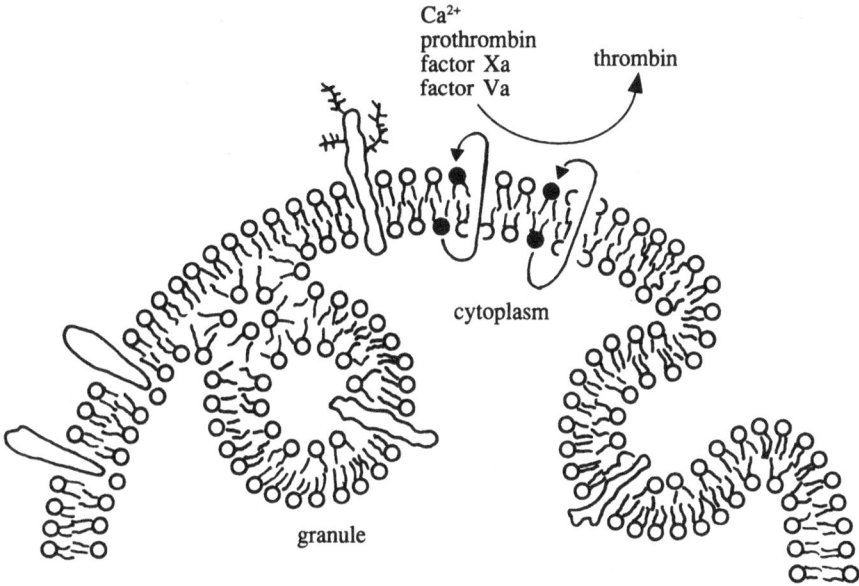

Fig. 18 The prothrombinase complex.

Upon platelet activation, phosphatidyl serine (●⟜) becomes exposed at the exterior of the surface membrane (here represented as a lipid bilayer with transmembrane and surface proteins). This triggers the interaction of prothrombin, calcium and factors Va and Xa (the prothrombinase complex) to form thrombin.

or collagen, a redistribution of phosphatidylserine occurs so that it becomes localised to the **outer** leaflet, at the platelet external surface, where the coagulation reactions can take place. This switch from one membrane leaflet to the other has been colloquially termed "flip-flop". It is intimately associated with the platelet cytoskeleton, which is "coupled" to the platelet plasma membrane and exerts a restraint to phospholipid transbilayer movement. The platelet agonists that are capable of eliciting platelet prothrombinase expression and thus initially phospholipid transbilayer movement, have been shown also to be able to activate a calcium-dependent protease, calpain, present in platelets. The amount of calpain activation correlates well with the amount of expression of prothrombinase at the platelet surface. It would seem that calpain cleaves particular cytoskeletal proteins, such as actin binding protein and myosin, and in so doing "uncouples" the cytoskeletal and membrane phospholipid restraining interactions thus facilitating transbilayer movement of phosphatidylserine.

A model of platelet prothrombinase activation thus envisages, upon their activation, stimulation of the enzyme calcium-dependent protease, which acts upon the cytoskeleton breaking the restraining hold it exerts upon the phospholipid surface, enabling transbilayer movement of these phospholipids, in turn resulting in increased expression of phosphatidylserine at the platelet surface. Phosphatidylserine is able to bind, via charge interactions, factors Xa, prothrombin and Va, in the presence of calcium to form thrombin. There is also good evidence that there exists a protein capable of inwardly transporting endogenous platelet phosphatidylserine back to the inner leaflet of the plasma membrane, thus completing the cycle.

Recent studies have implicated abnormalities in the above processes in certain disease states. For example, a patient has been described who presented with a bleeding disorder and was eventually found to have reduced platelet prothrombinase expression as a result of a possible aberration in the phosphatidylserine at the outer platelet membrane leaflet.

THE BERNARD-SOULIER SYNDROME

In this condition described by Bernard and Soulier in 1948, large platelets are observed, associated with prolonged bleeding times and haemorrhagic symptoms. It is an autosomal recessive disease, now thought to be the result of absent or defective platelet glycoprotein Ib and possibly also glycoprotein V, both of which are important cytoskeletal components, also involved in the binding of human factor VIII (von Willebrand factor) in turn important for the promotion of platelet agglutination responses. It is thought that the relative absence or defect in these platelet glycoproteins results in a reduction of the restraint exerted by the cytoskeleton upon phospholipid transbilayer movement and thus consequently enhanced basal expression of prothrombinase.

LUPUS

Systemic lupus erythematosus is an autoimmune disease affecting the skin, joints, kidneys, nervous system and mucous membranes, but in additon, it is associated with acquired inhibitors of coagulation. These lupus anticoagulants are principally immunoglobins of the IgG class, more rarely IgMs, which can predispose, paradoxically, to thrombosis. They are not necessarily confined to lupus but have also been found in other autoimmune diseases, following certain infections and drug treatments, e.g. of chlorpromazine, and also in some malignancies. What has become apparent is that purified lupus anticoagulants can react against negatively charged phospholipids such as phospatidylserine, phosphatidylinositol and cardiolipin. Indeed, as may be anticipated, recent work has shown that lupus anticoagulants can inhibit platelet prothrombinase activity by way of interaction with negatively charged phospholipids.

More work is needed to fully explore the interactions of platelet negatively charged phospholipids in other diseases, but at least this exciting field has highlighted the dynamic nature of cell membranes and the roles they play in biological systems. It adds an extra dimension to the concepts of membrane structure and function as described in the classical Singer/Nicholson fluid mosaic membrane model.

Further Reading

1. Bevers EM, Comfurius P and Zwaal RFA. Changes in membrane phospholipid distribution during platelet activation. *Biochim Biophys Acta* **736** : 57–66, 1983.
2. Galli M, Beguin S, Lindhout T and Hemker HC. Inhibition of phospholipid and platelet dependent prothrombinase activity in the plasma of patients with lupus anticoagulant. *Br J Haematol* **72** : 549–555, 1989.
3. Crook M. Platelet prothrombinase in health and disease. *Blood Coagulation and Fibrinolysis* **1** : 167–174, 1990.

5a

The Pill: Steroids Changing Shapes

If nothing else, the contraceptive pill generates superlative statistics — the most widely prescribed medication ever (aspirin of course does not need a prescription), one billion woman years of documented exposure to-date — with the social, economic and medical implications being no less immense. So steroid biochemistry, receptor affinity and feedback loops are highly important in the everyday lives of ordinary people after all.

It has been known for over eighty years that the corpus luteum is involved in the inhibition of ovulation during pregnancy. This pioneer study was later followed by clinical studies in which ovulation was inhibited by intramuscular oestradiol benzoate and later by oral noerthnodrel, a progestin (meaning a synthetic compound with progesterone-like activity). The problems with oestrogens and progesterone at this time were that (a) their actions were short-lived due to rapid hepatic inactivation *in vivo*, and (b) they were often inactive when taken by mouth due to poor absorption. So began the quest for synthetic compounds that would equal the endogenous ones in respect of biological response, duration of action, and acceptability by mouth. A reminder of the salient points of oestrogen synthesis is given in Fig. 19.

In the so-called combined pill — that is, containing both synthetic oestrogen and progestin — the commonly used oestrogens are ethinyloestradiol or its 3-methyl ether mestranol. (Stilboestrol was one of the first synthetic oestrogens but it was later found that substitution of the physiologically active compound oestradiol 17-β by adding a ethynyl group (carbon triple bond) at position 17 prolonged its activity. The oestrogen component of these pills inhibits ovulation by a central effect upon the hypothalamus, in turn suppressing release of follicle stimulating hormone (FSH) and luteinizing hormone (LH), which would normally trigger ovulation in mid-cycle.

The progestin constituent of the combined pill is usually a derivative of 19-nortesterone, i.e. testosterone without the methyl group at position 19. Examples are norgestrel, lynoestrenol, norethisterone, ethynodiol diacetate and norethynodrel. Another group of progestins are those derived from 17-hydroxyprogesterone,

cholesterol

↓

dehydroepiandrosterone

↓

androstenedione

testosterone   19-hydroxyandrostenedione

↓   ↓

19-hydroxytestosterone   oestrone

17 β-oestradiol

↓

oestriol

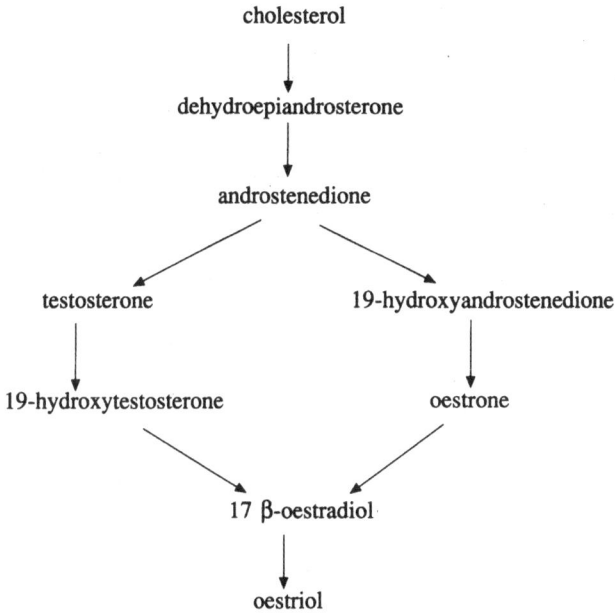

Fig. 19 Summary of oestrogen synthesis.

The synthesis of steroid hormones is perhaps unusual in that the end-products can often be achieved by alternative pathways. Also, in this summary an arrow does not necessarily represent a single reaction.

esterified at the 17-OH position, e.g. medroxyprogesterone acetate. Although nortesterone derivatives can be metabolised to oestrogen metabolites and thus exert an anti-ovulatory effect, progestins also confer a "pseudopregnant" state upon the endometrium and also increase cervical mucous thickness to impede penetration of spermatozoa.

Most modern pills consist of about 50 μg of oestrogen component, although the earlier versions contained at least three times this amount and were associated with a significant degree of oestrogen related side-effects. In addition modern oral contraceptives, rather than being fixed dose combinations, can now be prescribed in biphasic form, with a lower amount of progestin in the first ten days of the menstrual cycle. The strategy in part is an attempt more closely to mimic the physiological situation by facilitating endometrial proliferation during the first half of the menstrual cycle, which should in theory reduce the likelihood of break-through bleeding.

MINIS, TRIPHASICS AND DEPOTS

The so-called mini-pill contains only progestins, and although less effective than combined oral contraceptives, it can be used by women unable to tolerate the side effects of oestrogens; it can also be used by nursing mothers as lactation is not suppressed. Another method of modulating the dosages has been the introduction of triphasic pills which vary the amounts of synthetic oestrogen and progestin during the cycle in an effort to lower side-effects. It is the development of these which led some to say that the pill of 1990 has little resemblance whatsoever to that of 1960. Modes of administration have also expanded. Medroxyprogesterone acetate has been introduced subcutaneously in an oil solution (a depot injection) to suppress ovulation over several months.

IN THE SIDINGS

The side-effects of oral contraceptive agents, apart from their intrinsic clinical interest, yield insights into the actions of oestrogens and progestogens (this being the term for any natural progesterone-like substance), as well as being a useful aide-memoire for future prescribing.

The metabolic actions (which are by no means apparent, singly or collectively in **all** who use the pill) include:

(1) An increase in cholesterol and triglyceride in the plasma with norethisterone and laevonorgestrel-containing pills, for example, causing a decrease of high density lipoprotein (HDL), the so called cardioprotective lipoprotein fraction of the reverse cholesterol transport system (Chap. 4a).

(2) A rise in some of the blood clotting factors, such as   factor VII. Such observations may partly account for the   increased incidence of thromboembolic phenomena seen in a small but significant number of oral contraceptive users, particularly those who smoke or those taking a high dose oestrogen combination.

(3) The combined pill has also been shown to cause an increase in plasma renin substrate (see also Chap. 11c), which might in pārt explain the increased incidence of hypertension in some users.

(4) Some of the plasma transport proteins are increased, such as caeruloplasmin (a copper binding protein), transferrin (involved in iron regulation) and sex hormone and thyroid binding globulins. This last is relevant to plasma total thyroxine levels which are apparently raised because of this increase in the binding protein, although free thyroid hormone levels remain about normal.

(5) There is evidence that sometimes the combined preparations can block pyridoxine-dependent reactions causing the   breakdown of the essential

amino acid tryptophan (see also Chap. 16a). This is of interest as some users experience psychological depression that can sometimes be reversed by pyridoxine (that is vitamin B6) treatment.

(6) Other possible metabolic sequelae are a slight impairment in glucose tolerance, although there seems to be no increased risk of diabetes mellitus in normal women. It appears that a high progesterone potency could lower insulin binding to its receptor.

(7) A rare cholestatic jaundice has been documented in a very small number of users. This might be precipitated by the induction, in the liver, of catabolic enzymes.

More minor side-effects (albeit still troublesome) of these combined preparations are nausea, oedema, bloating, breast tenderness, chloasma (a suntan like coloration, principally of the face) and cyclic weight gain, all largely attributed to the oestrogen component. On the other hand acne, fatigue, decreased libido, shortened menstruation, and increased appetite are predominantly due to an excess of progestin.

Comment

The trade-off between the benefits of pregnancy avoidance and the often quite extensive side-effects are a matter of judgement for the clinician. A keen appreciation of the subtleties of the triphasics as exquisite biochemical modulators will make the task easier.

Further Reading

1. Steinberg WM. Oral contraception: risks and benefits *J Soc Obs Gyn Can* **12** : 9–15, 1990.
2. Shearin RB and Boehlke JR. Hormonal contraception. *Paed Clin N Amer* **36** : 695–715, 1989.

5b

The Price of Virility

When Ben Johnson was stripped of his gold medal after the 1988 Olympics, the general public acquired a nodding acquaintance with terms like **anabolic steroids** and **liver carcinoma**. Presumably superior strength and speed, and of course the bulging muscles, which make these abilities possible, have been the dream of many men and some women since the beginning of time. In the scientific era, it has been assumed that the greater muscle mass of males compared to females is due to testosterone and further, that increasing serum androgens above physiological levels will enhance muscle mass and thus athletic performance. Even in its infancy sports medicine took on a sinister dimension with reports of androgen use during the 1964 Tokyo Olympics, and the problem seemed to increase through the years, so much so that during the 1976 Montreal games, androgens were finally emplaced on the list of banned substances. Drug testing became mandatory in the 1984 Los Angeles Olympics.

ANDROGEN EFFECTS

In common with the other steroid hormones, androgens enter the target cell and interact with intracellular receptors, the hormone-receptor complex then enters the nucleus and interacts with chromosomal receptor sites, ultimately promoting gene transcription and synthesis of mRNA. This can result in a number of physiological actions, such as sexual differentiation, sexual maturation, regulation of gonadotrophin secretion, and increase in body weight. The separate androgenic and anabolic effects are consequent, not on different types of receptors, but on differential tissue expression of the stimulus. This is an important concept, since if confirmed it will render futile the attempts being made to develop drugs with "pure" anabolic actions, lacking androgen activity.

In the context of athleticism, there is evidence that muscles do have androgen receptors but the response is highly dependent upon the type of muscle group; however, in man it is reported that the muscles of the shoulder and pectoral girdle are particularly responsive. In this area androgenic steroids then probably promote the growth of new myofilaments and cause division of myofibrils, which is consistent with the increase in lean body mass seen in people using these drugs.

Testosterone is one of the principle physiological androgens but because of rapid first-pass metabolism, it cannot be effectively taken orally, and as administration by injection results in rapid metabolism, more long-acting derivatives of testosterone have been synthesised. (Note: this is exactly analogous to the problems involved in giving natural steroids as oral contraceptives.)

There are at least four main types of derivatives available for oral dosage:

(1) A pharmacological trick is to modify the testosterone molecule by alkylation at the 17-position with an ethyl or methyl group, which overcomes problems both of absorption and metabolism. Stanozolol and oxandrolone are examples.

(2) Another modification is alkylation at the position 1 of the steroid nucleus to give compounds like mesterolone.

(3) Esterification at the 17-position is yet another means of modifying testosterone, giving products an example of which is testosterone undecanoate.

(4) By esterification with carboxylic acids, the steroid molecule is made less polar and more soluble in lipid tissue, which causes a slower release of the compound into the circulation, an example being nandrolone. In a slightly different context, this may be of some clinical importance for the long-term treatment of male hypogonadism.

DO ANDROGENS DO THE TRICK?

Despite the foundation of biochemical knowledge noted above, some authorities have expressed doubts as to whether anabolic steroids in fact improve athletic performance and it would be ironic indeed, in view of the various athletic furores of the past few years, if it turned out ultimately to be all in the mind! The literature on the subject remains equivocal. However, it would only require a comparatively small increase in strength or speed to have considerable effects upon an athlete's performance at the topmost levels of sporting endeavour, wherein a fraction of a second may distinguish between a gold medal and second place, or a world record and comparative obscurity.

Although the benefits to athletic performance of androgenic steroids are hotly debated, there is less doubt regarding their potential harmful effects.

(1) Alkylated androgens can cause changes in liver function tests, such as the raising of serum alkaline phosphatase and unconjugated bilirubin, thus indicating hepatocellular damage.

(2) Further, this may be associated with the development of hepatoma and peliosis hepatitis, i.e. bloody cysts within the liver which possibly progress to hepatic carcinoma.

(3) Other metabolic effects include the lowering of high density lipoproteins, i.e the cardioprotective lipoprotein particle, and elevation of low density lipoproteins.

(4) Some power lifters taking large doses of androgens have been found to display impaired glucose tolerance and resistance to insulin.

(5) Obvious potential side-effects include virilising actions, such as acne, deepening of the voice, male pattern baldness and hirsutism seen in females.

(6) In males negative feedback control could result in the suppression of gonadotrophins, with subsequent decline in spermatogenesis. Indeed, such a mechanism has been proposed as the basis of male contraception. On top of this, testosterone and the other physiological androgen androstenedione are converted in extraglandular tissues to oestrogens such as oestradiol and oestrone. It is possible that synthetic androgens could be similarly converted. Thus, some male athletes on stacking regimes of androgen steroids have been found to exhibit gynaecomastia, a distinctly feminizing sign. (Or is this one way of "breasting" the tape earlier?)

The side-effects of androgen abuse are thus potentially large and varied. There is even an up-and-coming condition generated by success — the so-called Moscow syndrome wherein the muscle hypertrophy is so advanced that the ligaments and tendons, lagging behind, are inadequate for their mechanical tasks. *And* we do not have space here to discuss steroid induced psychosis, associated with two recent criminal trials for murder and attempted murder, of body builders in the United States.

NAILING THE CULPRIT

How can androgen abuse be detected? This demands much from the analyst-cum-detective who has to ensure discrimination of physiological levels of natural steroids from a variety of possible steroid culprits, possibly at very low levels. Suitable techniques include separation with gas or high pressure chromatography followed by identification using mass spectroscopy, for this combination can characterise steroids at concentrations as low as one part per billion, that is 1 nanogram in a gram. It is salutory to reflect that at the 1984 Los Angeles Olympics, of 1510 urines tested, 12 were positive for banned group anabolic steroids.

Testosterone esters form a difficult group of steroids to detect since, unlike some of the other synthetic steroids, they can be cleaved in the body to form testosterone which is then metabolised in the same way as endogenous testosterone. To attempt to overcome this problem, some workers have studied the changes in gonadotrophins which would be expected to decrease due to the feedback mechanism produced by an exogenous steroid. Others have concluded that exogenous testosterone is not epimerized to form epitestosterone to the same extent as endogenous sources, thus the testosterone/epitestosterone ratio can be taken as a an index of illicit dosage. The excretion of steroids can take place over a long time period, such as months. In efforts to evade detection, some abusers have tried to dilute excretion of these drugs by taking diuretics, e.g frusemide, while others have attempted to increase "washout" of the banned substances with agents such as probenecid, which probably acts upon the renal tubules.

It is obvious that, subliminal to the athletic contests proceeding on the track and field, there are other battles going on between sports physiologists/pharmacologists, possibly of unscrupulous bent, and organisers/officials backed up by analysts. Which of the two types of contest will be more keenly contested in the future is a moot point.

VIRILISING SYNDROMES

A heavy price is also paid by those suffering from the various endocrine disorders which lead to virilisation. The overt sign is the increased growth, not of the fine, or vellus type of hair which covers most surfaces of the body except the palms and soles, but the thicker terminal type on the face, trunk and extremities, for which androgens are entirely responsible. (They are even the stimulus for pubic and axillary hair in the female.) Causes of virilising syndromes are broadly classifiable as:

(1) Ovarian or adrenal tumours. Both these organs produce androgens and both can be the sites of secreting tumours.

(2) Polycystic ovary sundrome. There is also an overproduction of androgens in this condition, which involves infertility, and virilism. Its cause remains unknown.

(3) Congenital adrenal hyperplasia. If there is any blockage in the production of cortisol caused by enzyme deficiency, then feedback inhibition of ACTH secretion is diminished and hyperplasia of its target organ occurs. At the same time, the excessive production of pregnenolone leads not to cortisol but to alternative products. The most common deficiency resides with the 21α-hydroxylase which blocks both aldosterone and cortisol synthesis (Fig. 20). This leads to excessive production in the already hyperplastic gland of dehydroepiandrosterone and testosterone, with overt virilisation the extent of which depends upon the exact severity of the defect.

(4) Medication (minoxidil, diphenylhydantoin, penicillamine).

(5) Unknown (ethnicity, familial).

Logically, the therapy is to give female hormones (unless surgery is contemplated) conveniently in the form of oral contraceptive pills. Their efficacy is mediated by three mechanisms:

(1) The progestin component increases testostrone catabolism.

cholesterol
↓
pregnenolone   ⟶   dehydro-epiandrosterone
↓   ↓
progesterone   ⟶   androstenedione   ⟶   testosterone
↓   ↓
17α-hydroxy progesterone   oestrone   ⟶   17β-oestradiol

11-deoxy-corticosterone
↓
corticosterone
↓
aldosterone

11-deoxycortisol
↓
cortisol
↓
cortisone

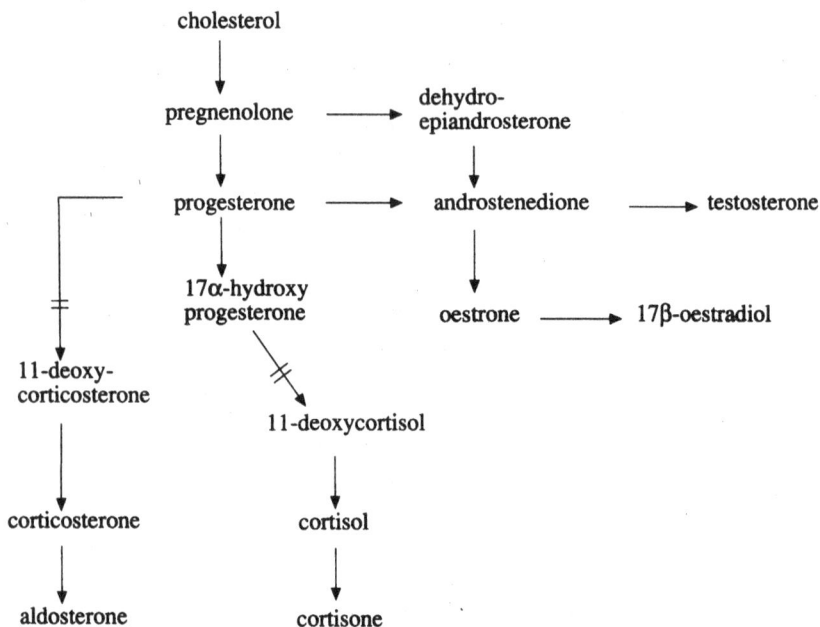

Fig. 20 Overview of corticoid hormone synthesis.

═ represents the block due to the 21-hydroxylase deficiency, the principal cause of congenital adrenal hyperplasia.

(2) The progestin component also suppresses luteinising hormone, which is a stimulus for testosterone secretion.

(3) The oestrogen component raises sex hormone binding globulin, which has the effect of sequestering testosterone in a biologically inactive form.

Contraception is desirable anyway to avoid the possibility of damage to a male foetus by the androgen blocking agents.

Further Reading

1. Park J, Park SJ, Lho DS, Choo HP, Chung B, et al. Drug testing at the 10th Asian games and 24th Seoul Olympic Games. *J Anal Toxicol* **14** : 66–72, 1990.
2. Erkkola R and Ruutiainen K. Hirsutism: definitions and aetiology. *Ann Med* **22** : 99–103, 1990.

5c
Old Bones

"No doubt there are many medical subjects which are far more exciting than old women with crumbling bones, and for the most part that is very much what osteoporosis is all about — or at least that is what we are given to believe."
— Dr Mark Aitken

There is a plausible sociobiological explanation for the menopause, related to the inordinate time, some 12–16 years, which it takes young human beings to attain an independent state. In default, had not evolutionary patterns settled on a termination of fertility some years before the end of the natural female lifespan, children born to women in the last years of their lives would have nobody to look after them. Hence the cessation of ovulation at about 50, when some years of active life, sufficient to nurture the last few offspring, can still be counted upon. Although the age at which the phenomenon occurs is said to be remaining fairly constant, since mean age expectancy is still rising in most countries, the postmenopausal fraction of their populations is increasing apace. If there are any associated clinical problems, then they can only become more important.

The "clock" which sets off the change is somewhere in the X-chromosome, and as it switches off oestrogen production from the ovary, the negative feedback inhibition on LH and FSH is cancelled. (Recall that at low levels of oestrogen there is a negative feedback on the gonadotrophins, but when critical concentrations are attained for a sufficient period then the feedback becomes positive instead, and they are synthesised in suffcient quantities to trigger ovulation.) Thus in older women enhanced FSH is likely to be a marker for diminishing secretion of oestrogen and it is easily measured in modern laboratories. (LH is a little different, requiring the polypeptide hormone inhibin for optimal secretion.)

Modern medical interest largely centres on the osteoporosis associated with oestrogen withdrawal. As opposed to osteomalacia, which is a preferential removal of bone mineral rather than matrix, osteoporosis involves resorption of both phases. The consequences are often fracture at a trabercular bone site such as the wrist, spine, or neck of the femur following an accident. Alternatively the patient may present with a backache due to vertebral compression.

The target tissues for oestrogens are naturally thought of as breast and uterus, and until recently it had been assumed that their influence on bone is indirect. Now, however, oestrogen receptors have been found on osteoblast-like cells from humans and mice, although their density is lower. The response of the cells appears to be to synthesise type I collagen, so age-related osteoporosis may well be a defect in the synthesis of matrix rather than mineral. However, others believe that it is basically a problem of calcium supply; osteoporotic women often have a demonstrable calcium malabsorption.

Be that as it may, obviously the problems consist in identifying those women at risk for osteoporosis, preventing it if possible, quantifying the degree of bone loss if it has already occurred, and conceivably, reversing the loss.

Care must also be taken to rule out other diseases which can cause bone loss and fractures, for example vitamin D deficiency, alcoholism, tumours, Cushing's syndrome, hyperthyroidism and hyperparathyroidism.

SERUM AND URINE CALCIUM

In the context of diagnosis, it has to be said that non-biochemical advances have been the most spectacular; dual photon absorptiometry, for instance, gives very rapid and reliable indices of bone mass. Risk assessment is being developed using predisposing factors, namely smoking and alcohol consumption, nulliparity, lack of exercise, calcium-poor diet, premature menopause or prolonged amenorrhea, and Caucasian or Asian race — these will generate a score indicating which subjects might be more intensively investigated. Women with osteoporosis usually have normal serum calcium and phosphate concentrations and also normal alkaline phosphatase activity, unless there has already been a fracture, when they will tend to be elevated. Marked hypercalcaemia in the absence of a fracture could be the result of hyperparathyroidism, bone metastases due to an occult tumour, or to multiple myeloma.

Urinary calcium, however, is of some diagnostic value, and if it is troublesome to collect a twenty-four hour specimen, the calcium/creatinine ratio can be calculated.

There are some promising indices of bone turnover involving bone matrix proteins, but they have not come into general use yet. Thus procollagen, the soluble precursor of matrix collagen, can be measured in serum, as can osteocalcin or Gla protein as the principal noncollagen protein produced by osteoclasts.

THERAPIES

All physicians will emphasise the importance of maintaining a good dietary supply of calcium, and moderate exposure to sunlight as an adjunct means of absorbing it through the good offices of vitamin D, especially if on account of the risk factors there seems the likelihood of osteoporosis before the menopause actually occurs. Oestrogen replacement therapy of course is now routine. For those who are thought to be at risk of thromboembolic disease, biphosphonates have been tried as an alternative; they are incorporated into bone mineral as it is laid down but block its removal by osteoclasts. Calcitonin has been given to some groups — its cost is high at the moment but a bioengineered supply should be available in due course.

Footnote

In a heroic study of almost nine thousand elderly Californian women, it has been shown that those with a history of oestrogen use had a 20% lower overall mortality than those who had never used them at all. The greater the period of use, the less seemed to be the overall mortality. The difference appeared to be due to the incidence of acute and chronic arteriosclerotic disease and cerebrovascular disease.

It is an interesting tie-up with the long-held belief that women in their reproductive years are protected, relative to their male counterparts, from arterial, including coronary arterial disease, by their ovaries.

Further Reading

1. Belchetz P. Endocrinology of the menopause. *The Practitioner* **234** : 491–493, 1990.
2. Riggs BL. A new option for treating osteoporosis. *N Eng J M* **323** : 124–1325, 1990.
3. Francis RM. If my wife had osteoporosis. *Br J Clin Pract* **43** : 109–112, 1989.
4. Henderson BE, Paganini-Hill and A Ross RK. Decreased mortality in users of oestrogen replacement therapy. *Arch Int Med* **151** : 75–78, 1991.

6a

Creatine Kinase: The Emergency Room Enzyme

With medical people intent on making the general public thoroughly knowledgeable about all aspects of heart disease, in the years ahead middle-aged men are liable to deliver themselves in ever greater numbers to the emergency centre if they experience chest pains. "Chest pain" however is a subjective matter, and a second member of the triad for detecting myocardial infarction, namely electrocardiography, is usually employed without delay. But this too can give ambiguous information and the third, the creatine kinase (CK) activity in the serum, really comes into its own.

ENZYMES AND ENERGY IN MUSCLES

We all first meet CK as the enzyme catalysing the reaction:

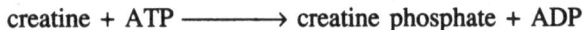

$$\text{creatine} + \text{ATP} \longrightarrow \text{creatine phosphate} + \text{ADP}$$

in the interests of maintaining a pool of energy-producing substrate in the myocyte. The equilibrium is such that there are about equal amounts of ATP and creatine phosphate in the muscles, but if ATP is used up the reserve of creatine phosphate is sufficient only for 2–3 sec of intense muscular activity. Glycolysis soon accelerates after the creatine phosphate is exhausted and restores the supply of ATP (plus the rather less benign lactic acid).

CK however is found in most tissues, if in smaller amounts than in muscle. There are quite large concentrations, though, in tissues such as urinary bladder and uterus. This would seem a disadvantage in the use of it for diagnostic purposes, but of course an experienced clinician is not going to confuse a disorder of the urinary bladder with that of muscle, whatever the enzymes tell him.

CREATINE KINASE ISOENZYMES

A further way of distinguishing the heart from the other forms of the enzyme is by isoenzyme identification. CK isoenzymes, which as usual are most conveniently separated one from another by electrophoresis, are thankfully simple. There are two subunits, coded for by different structural genes, designated B (for brain) and M (for muscle) which are associated in the intact molecule as dimers. Two units can combine in only three ways, that is the three CK isoenzymes are BB, MB and MM. (They were subsquently renamed CK-1, CK-2 and CK-3 respectively when the clinical chemistry bureaucracy took an interest, a nomenclature not nearly as easy to remember; it is based on electrophoretic mobility.) The CK-MB can now be rapidly and accurately estimated in clinical laboratories by eliminating the MM with specific antibodies and estimating the remaining CK activity, that is MB. (Unless there is reason to believe that there may be brain damage or certain cancers, the possibility of a rise in CK-BB is discounted.)

OTHER ENZYMES AND HEART ATTACK

Usually, **parallel** testing, that is measuring two or more different indices of a disease at the same time, increases diagnostic **sensitivity**, which here has the special technical meaning of the probability of detecting that disease when the patient is in fact and reality suffering from it. There are a number of other enzymes available for the detection of damage to heart muscle, but only two have held their ground, namely lactate dehydrogenase (LDH) and aspartate aminotransferase (AST). The argument against parallel testing is that it tends to increase the number of false positives, that is, it is not so good for **excluding** disease — also it increases costs.

AST and LDH activities do not increment at the same rate in serum — they are released from the necrotic tissue at the same time certainly, but their rise is a reflection of the amount of activity originally present in the cells; the subsequent fall, moreover, is a reflection of the half-life of the enzymes in the serum (Fig. 21). That is why, if a patient comes in for assessment at about 48 hours after the suspected cardiac episode, a falling AST and LDH may yet point to an infarct when CK is already again normal.

CLINICAL CONUNDRUM

A forty-six-year old executive came into the the emergency department complaining of severe chest pain, radiating to the back. He had tolerated it for an hour or two, but was then forced to seek help. When seen he was distressed, pale sweating, and breathless. He was also coughing a lot, and this had started at the onset of the pains. On examination heart sounds were normal, and no murmurs were heard. However there was tachypnoea with very minimal movement of the chest wall. Questioning elicited that he had been asthmatic for six years and was on maintenance doses of steroids. The principal possibilities were thought to be:

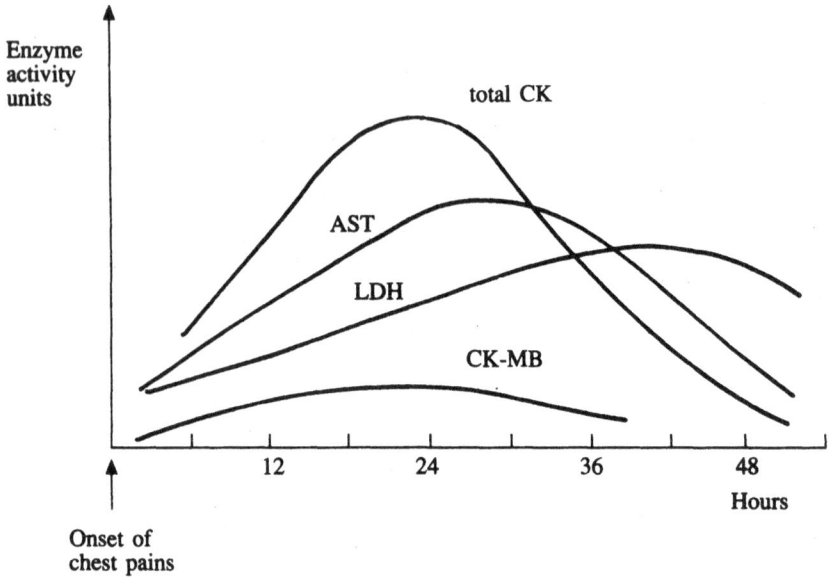

Fig. 21   Course of serum enzyme activities after myocardial infarction.

AST = aspartate transminase   LDH = lactic dehydrogenase
CK = creatine kinase. CK-MB is not normally detected in the serum. The relative rise and
fall of the enzyme activities depends not only on the course of the infarct but on the methods
used for measuring the activities.

(1) Myocardial infarction with pulmonary oedema.
(2) Dyspepsia as a consequence of steroid therapy.
(3) A collapsed dorsal vertebra due to steroidoigenic osteoporosis.
(4) Spontaneous pneumothorax (rupture of the pleura with air entering the chest,
     as a result of the asthma).

Further questioning elicited that he had taken an antacid tablet, which however
had failed to relieve the pain, and this does tend to rule out number 2 above.
Moreover, breathlessness is normally unlikely to derive from oesophagitis, the
burning sensation in the gullet due to the dyspepsia. Number 3 was considered
unlikely in that there was no aggravation of the pain by movement of the spine.

While further investigations were being arranged (ECG, chest X-ray, and blood
chemistries) he was given intramuscular diamorphine for the pain, then intramuscular frusemide (a diuretic) to relieve the highly probable pulmonary oedema. He

became more comfortable, and the results began to come in. The ECG appeared to be normal, and the X-ray allowed elimination of pneumothorax, although it did demonstrate a definite pulmonary oedema. The blood chemistry was unremarkable except for a moderately raised total CK. On the basis that a heart attack was very probable, anticoagulation and reperfusion therapy was almost instituted, when a further lab result, after CK isoenzyme typing (a little delayed beyond the result for the total enzyme activity since the laboratory had to do an incubation step) showed that the rise was due to CK-MM. CK-MB remained at the normal level of under 5% of the total. Here is a dilemma! How can there be a heart attack if the CK-MB does not rise? But it is easy to be deceived — somebody then remembered the injections and the coughing. These can cause quite marked rises in total CK, the enhanced activity residing in the muscle form, MM, not MB. (In this case the injections were probably too recent to raise CK-MM, and so blame must be ascribed to the coughing). The only thing to do was to take more blood at four and eight hours and indeed the total and CK-MB, as well as AST started to rise steeply. It was concluded that indeed he had indeed had a heart attack and appropriate therapy was instituted without delay.

Comment

The case shows that (1) the enzymes can be critical for diagnosis; (2) the isoenzyme patterns are especially informative; and (3) you have to give the enzyme activities time to rise in the serum before being sure about the diagnosis. Another test which is coming into prominence and can be applied very early after the infarct is serum myoglobin — this is a very early indicator of damage to heart muscle, because it is released into the circulation early by virtue of its low molecular weight. It is conveniently detected by its reaction with an antibody bound to latex particles — if it is present the latex agglutinates on a slide, rather as seen in the well-known pregnancy tests. The myoglobin test is almost one hundred percent, specific, that is it is excellent for **excluding** myocardial infarction, for the period up to about twelve hours after the chest pains were experienced.

Further Reading

1. Leung F Y, Galbraith L V, Jablonsky G and Henderson A R. Re-evaluation of the diagnostic utility of serum total creatine kinase and creatine kinase-2 in myocardial infarction. *Clin Chem* **35** : :1435–1444, 1989.
2. Jones M G and Swaminathan R. The clinical biochemistry of creatine kinase. *J Int Fed of Clin Chem* **2**, 108–115, 1990.

6b

Lactase and the Milky Way

When is an enzyme deficiency a disease? Does it have to produce a distinct pathology, like the mental retardation of phenylketonuria consequent upon phenylalanine
hydroxylase deficiency? What if the manifestations only appear upon challenge, as
in the case of a lack, or variant of, glucose 6-phosphate dehydrogenase? If the
pathology is manifested in the majority of the world's population only upon
challenge by some unusual and adverse circumstance, is it a disease? Obviously the
answer has to be "no". But lactase deficiency, which comes into this last category,
was thought to be a disease for a long time. It had been noticed by some Western
physicians travelling or working in the tropics that many non-Europeans, upon
being given milk to drink, developed a series of gastrointestinal symptoms, like
nausea, bloating, stomach cramps, flatulence and diarrhoea. This constellation was
thought to be psychogenic since for these people milk was such an unusual food —
the situation is rather analogous to the nausea and vomiting you might expect in an
Englishman induced to eat dog meat. About 1960 the investigation of the phenomenon of milk intolerance was put on a scientific basis by Dalquist and others, who
showed that the symptoms were due to lactose ("milk sugar") and who developed
a lactose tolerance test. If the lactose is not absorbed, it passes into the large bowel
where bacteria ferment it to methane, hydrogen, and fatty acids which make the
stools quite acidic. The hyperosmolality of the colonic fluid causes diarrhoea and
the gases cause the flatulence and bloating. The test developed in the sixties was
similar to the glucose tolerance test, but assesses ability to absorb the substance
from the diet rather than to assimilate it into the tissues. Nowadays breath hydrogen
instead of blood glucose is usually measured after the lactose challenge — indeed
breath hydrogen is a useful index of quite a few malabsorption syndromes. In any
case, putting one test or another into practice enabled a survey of which populations
were lactase deficient, and which ones could drink milk. It turned out this way:

Deficient: South Italians, Turks, Ethiopians, Kalahari Bushmen, Moroccans,
Chinese at home and abroad, Japanese, Vietnamese, Indonesians, South Indians,
New Guineans, Eskimos, Southern Sudanese.

Tolerant: Northern Europeans and their emigre extensions (Americans, Canadi-
ans, Australians, etc.), Bedouin Arabs, North Indians, Tuaregs, Northern Sudanese.

Very few of these populations gave a 100% response one way or another, but one or two did, e.g. the Vietnamese and the Japanese. So it turns out that most of the world's population (the inclusion of the Chinese alone in the first of the lists above guarantees this fact) are unable to digest lactose in adult life, and thus to drink milk. However they can take other milk products. Cream, being the fatty supernatant of milk after it is boiled or left to stand, has no lactose, and in cheese and yoghurt the lactose is almost entirely consumed by the microorganisms responsible for the flavour and taste of the finished product. But why is lactose in the milk in the first place?

WHY LACTOSE?

The mammary gland has a finely-tuned system for synthesising lactose for the nutrition of the infant. It depends upon the enzyme uridine diphosphogalactosyl epimerase, which converts a glucose molecule to uridine diphosphogalactose (UDP-galactose), then upon a transferase which links up this to another molecule of glucose. The transferase only acts if it comes into contact with the protein α-lactalbumin, the gene for the synthesis of which is switched on by prolactin from the pituitary. It is switched off again by progesterone, when ovulation and formation of the corpus luteum is resumed. The transferase also occurs in other tissues, where it participates in the synthesis of glycoproteins; somehow its specificity is altered in the breast tissue when it interacts with α-lactalbumin, such that it binds glucose and the UDP-galactose instead, with lactose as the final product. But why synthesise this molecule, when, as the diagram (Fig. 22) shows, the livers of young mammals, like those of the old, have to convert galactose released in the gastrointestinal tract back to glucose if this carbohydrate source of energy is to be utilised at all? The answer presumably lies in a sort of metabolic altruism. Nowhere in the mother's tissues (the lumen of the duodenum is another matter — that is really outside the body) is there a lactase. She has no means of breaking it down again for her own energy needs should the necessity arise — it is purely for export, for the survival of the offspring.

WHY MILK?

Although almost any material containing protein, fat or carbohydrate can be consumed by human beings, some might indeed see the ingestion of the secretion of the mammary gland, a fluid designed for the temporary sustenance of very young animals, as bizarre. It is certainly unusual, in that most of the world's population fundamentally lack the capacity to digest it. And there is probably a survival value attached here too. Man as a species came into existence about one and a half million years ago (mammals *per se* a long time before that) and life must have been fairly

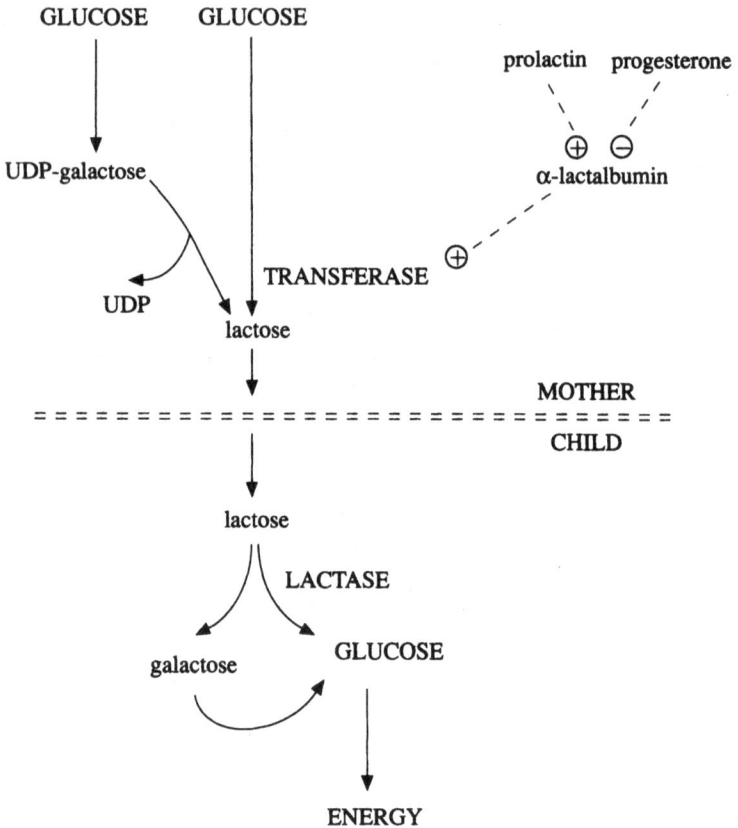

Fig. 22 The synthesis (by the mother) and exploitation (by the infant) of lactose.

The upper part summarises the synthesis in the mammary gland, the lower the assimilation into the baby's tissues after it is hydrolysed to galactose and glucose in the duodenum. Before the birth, the hormone progesterone from the ovary switches off the synthesis of α-lactalbumin, which is potentially able to direct the mammary gland to synthesise lactose rather than other products. At parturition, progesterone is overcome by prolactin from the pituitary and α-lactalbumin and therefore lactose is synthesised. The whole process begins and ends with glucose. The complicated synthesis of lactose from it provides a carrier of energy which cannot be utilised by the mother, but which the baby can cope with due to the intestinal lactase.

precarious for the naked, two-legged, slow moving individuals who emerged. Forcible if not rapacious uplifting of the nutritious secretion of the mammary gland of nursing mothers in the cave must often have seemed an attractive alternative to the dangers of the hunt, even to the exhausting competition with hyenas for carrion. Of course, if greedy adults had been able to steal and digest this milk, the tribe would have died out. There had to be some constraint, namely the unpleasant effects of lactose malabsorption.

But somehow, despite this constraint, the adult lactase gene did evolve. Some advantage in its presence outweighed the dangers outlined above. The fact that, by and large, it only survived in populations living in temperate climates suggests that it had something to do with the migration northwards of the first hominids, who had their ultimate origins in Africa. It is possible that these migrants took domesticated animals with them as they drove nothwards, and gradually learned to milk them as they left their established food supplies. But it turns out that milk sugar has a very valuable property — it aids in the absorption of calcium. As humans ventured further from the sunlight of the equator they became more at risk from vitamin D deficiency. They developed lighter skins to absorb more of the sunlight that was available, true, but they also began to drink milk containing lactose, which by aiding calcium absorption circumvented much of the external requirement for the vitamin.

CHOLERA, RATHER?

Gordon Cook has pointed out that the adult lactase gene developed in areas which have never been devoid of sunlight, such as the Arabian Peninsula and the Punjab, and suggested that the Bedouins and Punjabis developed the adult lactase gene to allow milk drinking as a protection against cholera. In the first place this would make available a sterile sodium and potassium-rich fluid (these ions are very much depleted in cholera due to their loss from the gastrointestinal tract during the profuse diarrhoea) but additionally, milk appears to prevent the growth of bacteria in the human small intestine, possibly due to a protein called lactoferrin.

There is one other interesting aspect to all of this. All nutritionists will tell you that milk is poor in iron (despite the lactoferrin); babies in general are born with enough iron stores to see them through the suckling period but reliance on milk alone for too long will result in a partial iron deficiency. It turns out however that partial iron deficiency produces a resistance to infections, such as malaria and tuberculosis; a sufficiency of iron in the blood is presumably necessary for parasitic replication. The adult lactase gene is therefore a powerful survival advantage if it promotes milk drinking to this effect also.

CLINICAL APPLICATIONS

Lactose intolerance is similar to the alcohol flushing syndrome (Chap. 18c) in being an apparent anthropological curiosity, but it has some important clinical implications. There are suggestions that heart disease is linked to lactose consumption; they are based on epidemiological studies, which cannot be taken up in a biochemistry book. Of more substance is the connection between lactose and cataracts. After galactose is absorbed, it is metabolised by the liver to galactose 1-phosphate, preparatory to oxidation. If there is a persistent galactose excess however, the lens of the eye converts galactose, by means of the enzyme aldose reductase, to galactitol, sometimes also known as dulcitol. This enzyme also reduces glucose, but has less affinity for it than it has for galactose. So surges of galactose cause accumulation of galactitol, leading to hyperosmolality in the lens, and eventual opacity. Galactitol is not removed by sorbitol dehydrogenase, as is sorbitol. In summary:

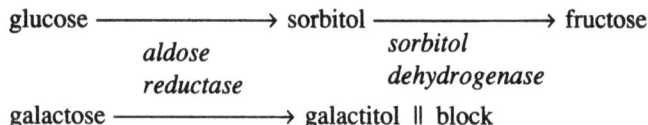

glucose —————————→ sorbitol —————————→ fructose
         aldose   *sorbitol*
         reductase   *dehydrogenase*
galactose —————————→ galactitol ‖ block

Thus so-called senile cataracts may possibly be engendered by decades of milk drinking. Whether to advise people to forego the obvious nutritional value of milk (if they are lactose tolerant) to avoid possible opacities in old age is a question not easy to answer.

But finally, on a very practical level:

(1) If you are working with refugees, try to find out if they have been accustomed to milk drinking before accepting dried milk as the main relief food. In any case, give them small amounts of reconstituted milk to start with, to see how well they tolerate it.

(2) If you know you are working with population low in adult lactase, try giving a big glass of milk to any patient for whom you want an inexpensive laxative.

Further Reading

1. Cook GC. Primary and secondary hypolactasia, Chap. 21. In: *Tropical Gastroenterology*. Oxford University Press, 1980.
2. Flatz G. The genetic polymorphism of intestinal lactase activity in adult humans, Chap. 122. In: Scrivver CL, ed. *The metabolic basis of inherited disease*, 6th ed. 19.

PART TWO

Metabolic Patterns and their Perturbations

7a
Lactic Acidosis

Lactic acidosis is a common medical emergency. It cannot be considered a disease in itself, of course, any more than jaundice or hyperlipidaemia, in themselves, are diseases. It is rather the manifestation of a number of syndromes and lesions (although it does appear in *Disease a Month*, Ref. 1 below). Lactic acid was a difficult substance to quantitate in blood until the modern era, but when a large number of measurements from various types of patients became available about thirty years ago, Huckabee realised that he could distinguish two types of lactic acidosis, A and B. The classification was made more complex afterwards and, in an unprecedented move, simplified again in the spirit of the original very clear distinction. Lactic acidosis type A is simply due to poor tissue perfusion of oxygen, and B is due to a large number of causes which do not appear to include, at least initially, a hypoxic component. The simple subdivisions of the latter are:

    B1 — miscellaneous,
    B2 — poisons,
    B3 — hereditary enzyme deficiencies.

GLYCOLYSIS YET AGAIN

Lactic acid is the end product of glycolysis, but is minimally produced when oxygen flux through tissues is normal. In serum it is usually less than 1 mmol/l. This is because its precursor, pyruvate, is mostly channelled into the citric acid cycle when there is a plentiful supply of oxidised nucleotides (principally NAD). When it is produced in great quantities by rapidly exercising muscle subject to "oxygen debt", it reaches the liver in the systemic circulation and is synthesised to glycogen there. This is the Cori cycle — a cycle because of course once within the liver the carbon atoms are available for release once again as glucose for reutilisation by the muscles.

    Build-up of lactic acid causes a metabolic acidosis, because a neutral substance, namely glucose, has been converted into a substance which ionises.

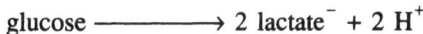

$$\text{glucose} \longrightarrow 2 \text{ lactate}^- + 2 \text{ H}^+$$

When lactate is oxidised to carbon dioxide and water, the stoichiometry demands that two hydrogen ions be removed again.

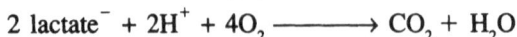

$$2 \text{ lactate}^- + 2H^+ + 4O_2 \longrightarrow CO_2 + H_2O$$

It does not particularly matter at what stage in the oxidation process the protons become available, or where they derive from. If there is a surge of lactic acid, there is inevitable acidosis; when the lactate is removed, the acidosis is cancelled. Whether in lactic acidosis the lactate ion itself is harmful, or whether the damage is done by the hydrogen ions themselves, is a question which has not been finally settled. There is a clue however, from panic attacks. Sodium lactate infusions reliably induce panic in patients who are prone to such attacks, but not in normal controls. This cannot be due to acidosis, for administration of the sodium salt is quite different from that of the acid. This can be seen, once again, by writing out the reaction for the metabolic disposal.

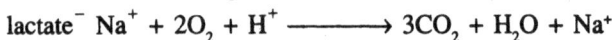

$$\text{lactate}^- \text{ Na}^+ + 2O_2 + H^+ \longrightarrow 3CO_2 + H_2O + Na^+$$

So sodium lactate simply mops up protons during its oxidation; it cannot contribute them — in fact it produces alkalosis rather than the reverse. The panic attacks could conceivably be due to alkalosis if the loss of acid is not compensated for quickly; it could also be due to the lactate ion itself. However, there may be other reasons, such as sequestering of calcium ions by the lactate anion, to the detriment of anxiolytic neurones.

A AND B

A breakdown of types A and B lactic acidosis is as follows:

Type A
(1) Respiratory failure
(2) Anaemias
(3) Shock

These are evidently conditions in which supply of oxygen to tissues is inadequate. It is easy enough to rationalise the emplacement of the first two within type A, but shock is often reported in the media as a sort of non-specific response to an accident. It is in fact a syndrome involving hypotension and tachycardia as a result of blood loss, septicaemia, or poor cardiac function (cardiogenic shock). Septic shock is a systemic response to infection and inflammation. Cardiogenic shock results from myocardial infarction as a natural consequence of the failure of the heart as a pump. Shock may also be psychogenic, as after emotional trauma.

Type B
B1 (1) Muscle damage
(2) Thiamine deficiency
(3) Leukaemias and other tumours
(4) Liver diseases

(5) Exercise
B2 (1) Poisons (ethanol, methanol, ethylene glycol, salicylates)
    (2) Fructose
B3 Various enzyme deficiencies
        — glycogen storage diasease
        — fructose 1,6-diphosphatase
        — mitochondrial defects

This is a formidable list, but many of the items are dealt with in other sections (poisoning in Chap. 13a; muscle damage in 12a; alcohol in 18c; thiamine in 15b; fructose in 2b). We also mention, though do not explain, the lactic acidosis of a number of inherited diseases of metabolism in Chap. 9a.

It is a moot point as to whether exercise should be classed as type A (too little oxygen for too much muscle activity) or type B (muscle damage due to stress and hypoxia), or maybe since it is essentially non-pathological, it should not be in the list at all. However, it is the cause of stiffness after heavy exercise, and perhaps part of the pain during it.

The enzyme deficiencies which cause lactic acidosis are many and varied, and may give the most severe problems in diagnosis; in the end, the suspect enzyme may have to be measured in a suitable cell, such as the hepatocytes of a liver biopsy. Below is an example of such an investigation.

A CHINA-DOLL CASE

A two year old girl was brought to the clinic by her parents because they noticed her abdomen becoming progressively more distended. It was established that the liver was 13 cm below the costal margin so that it could be described as a gross hepatomegaly. Some preliminary blood chemistry was done, and showed the following:

glucose	—	1.2 mmol/l	(normal, 4–7.8)
lactic acid	—	5.2 mmol/l	(< 2.5)
uric acid	—	610 μmol/l	(180–410)
triglyceride	—	3.7 mmol/l	(0.5–2.0)
cholesterol	—	6.1 mmol/l	(<5)

Immediately, this was almost diagnostic of glycogen storage disease, especially since the child, on close scrutiny, had the china doll-like face which is typical thereof. The hypoglycaemia is due to the inability of the liver to recycle glucose units through glycogen; the hyperuricaemia to the wastage of ATP (see Chap. 3d), the hyperlipidaemia to the efforts of the body to mobilise fats as substrates in the absence of adequate energy from blood glucose. Meanwhile the liver is swelling up with non-utilisable glycogen granules and also fat mobilised to it. But which of the glycogenoses is this exactly? Types I and III (glucose 6-phosphatase and amylo-1,6-glucosidase deficiency respectively) show the same sort of pattern and physical appearance. Types V and VII are diseases of skeletal muscle and may be readily excluded. The remaining types tend to be either mild or fatal quite early in life, not intermediate as in the child seen in this case.

A glucagon stimulation test was done. Glucagon, of course, activates phosphorylase, which begins the degradation of glycogen by removing successive glucose units, as glucose 1-phosphate, from the ends of the branches in the molecule. In the case of type I, the glucose 1-phosphate is converted to glucose 6-phosphate satisfactorily, but blood sugar cannot be augmented due to the lack of the phosphatase. Nonetheless, some glucose is formed, for the amylo-1,6-glucosidase, also known as debranching enzyme, renoves the glucose stub after the action of the transferase (Fig. 23); in type III there is generally no increase in blood sugar after the glucagon stimulus; the lack of the glucosidase means that removal of glucose units from the large glycogen granules is minimal, for it always stops at a branch point. In the case of the child under investigation, the figures for the test were:

Time	Glucose, mmol/l	Lactate, mmol/l
0 (fasting)	4.5	12.4
30	5.5	14.9
45	5.7	15.1

So this is type I or von Gierke's disease. There is a small increase in glucose, but a marked extra surge of lactate as glycolysis is further stimulated by the glucose phosphates made available by glycogenolysis. Complete confirmation was by assaying the enzyme in a liver biopsy.

Treatment of type I is not very satisfactory but this child was given a corn starch diet. This effects a slow release of glucose into the portal circulation, to minimise glycogen synthesis in the liver and the associated hepatomegaly.

TUMOURS AND LACTIC ACIDOSIS

It has been known for some time that leukaemia sufferers have a lactic acidosis. This may be due to:
(1) Lactate production by the massive numbers of leukocytes in the circulation.
(2) Tissue hypoxia due to blockage of small blood vessels by aggregations of leukocytes.
(3) Impaired liver function in leukaemia.

Dr McConnel (Ref. 3 below) reports a case of the young woman who was feeling generally ill, with dyspnoea. She had always been in good health except for a breast

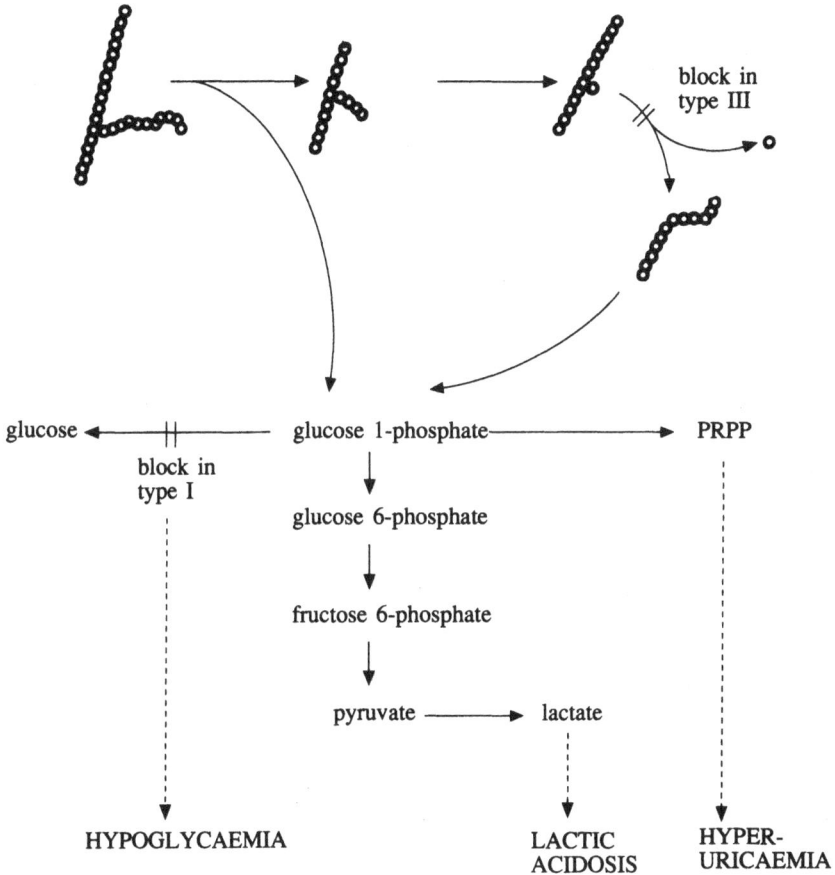

PRPP = 5-phosphoribosylpyrophosphate
  o = glucose units in the dextrans

Fig. 23 Summary of glycogen metabolism in relation to glycogenoses types I and III.

Glycogen is converted to limit dextran with four-unit stubs, after which a transferase removes a trisaccharide and attaches it to a free end, leaving a dextran with single 1,6-linked glucosyl units. If amylo-1-6-glucosidase is lacking as in glycogenosis type III the process stops at that point and hypoglycaemia results. In type I where the glucose 6-phosphatase is lacking, formation of glucose for the maintenance of euglycaemia is blocked, and the enhanced alternative pathways tend to produce lactic acidosis and hyperuricaemia.

lump some months previously, which proved to be an invasive adenocarcinoma, and a right mastectomy had been performed. When she came into hospital on the latter occasion, she was noted to be shocked and tachypnoeic, with a high pulse rate and a blood pressure so low it could not be measured. She was given a pressor drug immediately. Some blood sent to the laboratory for STAT chemistries showed lactate to be extremely high, at 16 mmol/l. Since lactic acidosis is often caused by poisons, there was close questioning to try to eliminate this. The doctors also strongly suspected septic shock, but could not pin down any infection despite strenuous efforts. The other possible differential diagnosis was lactic acidosis type B, but as we have learned so far, this hardly takes one further than the provision of a label since its components are so diverse. Unfortunately, despite antibiotic therapy as a preemptive strike against the still possible sepsis, the patient deteriorated and died within a few hours.

What had happened? The autopsy told the story. As a result of the breast cancer, she had metastases in the lymph nodes, two lower thoracic vertebrae, and the liver. No infection could be found. Thus, solid tumours can also cause lactic acidosis. First of all, they can conduct a vigorous glycolysis which will produce the acid; moreover, if the liver is impaired it cannot be removed. Here the shock was caused by the acidosis, not the reverse. The case also illustrates that a high lactic acid on presentation (like a high urate, Chap. 3d) is an indicator of poor chance of survival.

Comment

Lactic acidosis crops up many times throughout these pages. This is not because of any obsession but because, as a pathological marker, it is seen in such a vast range of diseases. More, it is the epitome of metabolic medicine, in that basic biochemical knowledge allows a thorough understanding of its pathogenesis and treatment. That is sufficient excuse.

Further Reading

1. Mizock BA. Lactic acidosis *Disease-a-month*, April, 1989.
2. Cohen RD and Woods HF. Lactic acidosis revisited. *Diabetes* **32** : 181–191, 1983.
3. McConnel AA, Parfitt VJ and Walker PR. An unusual case of shock in a young woman. *Postgrad Med J* **65** : 120, 1989.
4. Liebowitz MR, Gorman JM, Fyer AB, et al. Lactate provocation of panic attacks. *Arch Gen Psychiatry* **42** : 709–719, 1985.

7b

Hypoglycaemia

Early in 1990, a world distressed about the fate of the hostages in Lebanon was relieved to see one of them, Robert Polhill, emerge from his long captivity. He was a little uncoordinated and his voice was rather flat; but the most noticeable characteristic was his extreme leanness, for he had been half-starved. It later emerged that he was diabetic. It must have occurred to all those interested in metabolism that, as a diabetic without access to medical care, the starvation had possibly saved Robert Polhill's life. Before the insulin era, starvation was the only treatment for diabetes mellitus; it forced a degree of hypoglycaemia on the sufferer, whereas on the contrary the provision of square meals risked postprandial hyperglycaemia, ketosis, acidosis, and coma. It was a drastic therapy for patients who had usually suffered severe weight loss from the disease in the first place. But insulin became available in the twenties and the oral hypoglycaemics, the sulphonylureas, in the fifties, and starvation could be replaced, as one of the salient means of therapy, by mere restriction of sugary foods.

CAUSES OF HYPOGLYCAEMIA

Vincent Marks says there are over one hundred different causes of hypoglycaemia, defined as a serum glucose of 2.5 mmol/l or less. Starvation is only the most basic of them. Some of the others are as follows:

(1) Reactive hypoglycaemia
(2) Insulinoma
(3) Hypopituitarism
(4) Liver disease
(5) Alcohol
(6) Tumours
(7) Infections
(8) Inherited disorders — glycogen storage disease
galactosaemia

As causes of hypopglycaemia, most of these are easy enough to explain. Deficiency of growth hormone or ACTH will tend to allow hypoglycaemia, for both are insulin antagonists (the latter via cortisol). Some tumours appear to release a factor with insulin-like activity. Infections cause an enhanced requirement for energy as glucose, and so a situation akin to starvation can arise if stores of glycogen are inadequate. The liver, as the main producer of glucose from its glycogen stores, must remain patent for the maintenance of euglycaemia. Alcohol produces hypoglycaemia in fasting subjects by trapping gluconeogenic substates as lactate but it may also affect the liver (Chap. 18c). The inherited causes are dealt with elsewhere (Chap. 7a). The two remaining are discussed below.

The symptoms of hypoglycaemia are sweating, tachycardia, anxiety, clamminess of the skin, sometimes nausea and vomiting, because the low glucose concentration triggers a sympathomedullary response, involving secretion of adrenaline.

REACTIVE HYPOGLYCAEMIA

At the top of the list above is one of the most interesting causes of hypoglycaemia, in that it may not really exist, or if it does, its prevalence is minute. This is **reactive** — sometimes known as **rebound** — hypoglycaemia. Another name is **functional hypoglycaemia**. Since the symptoms of hypoglycaemia are non-specific and non-diagnostic, the idea grew up that all sorts of vague feelings of ill-health, depression or anxiety could be ascribed to it. There is no doubt that in some people the secretion of insulin after a meal pushes the blood glucose to below the basal, preprandial level (Fig. 24) but the vogue which developed for a self-diagnosed illness led to an unprecendented joint admonition from the American Medical Association, the Endocrine Society, and the American Diabetes Association. There was no evidence, they said, that hypoglycaemia, even if it occurred in some subjects, was linked to depression, chronic fatigue, allergies, nervous breakdown, juvenile delinquency, or inadequate sexual performance. So that is that!

Where it is an established phenomenon, it is evidently due to an imbalance between glucose availability and utilisation, involving the persistence of glucose uptake by insulin sensitive tissues, including the liver in a glycogenetic mode.

HUMAN INSULIN

Everybody in the street outside knows that diabetes is a disease of high blood sugar, but those who study metabolic medicine have to recognise that the reverse situation, hypoglycaemia, is a recurrent problem in diabetics. It is caused, of course, by an overdose of insulin or the relevant oral medication. Until a few years ago, the preparation which diabetics were taught to inject was pig insulin, which was thought however not to be ideal, since it differs from human in one amino acid residue. Indeed it can slowly elicit antibodies in some patients. Improvement was sought and human insulin was the first molecule produced by recombinant DNA

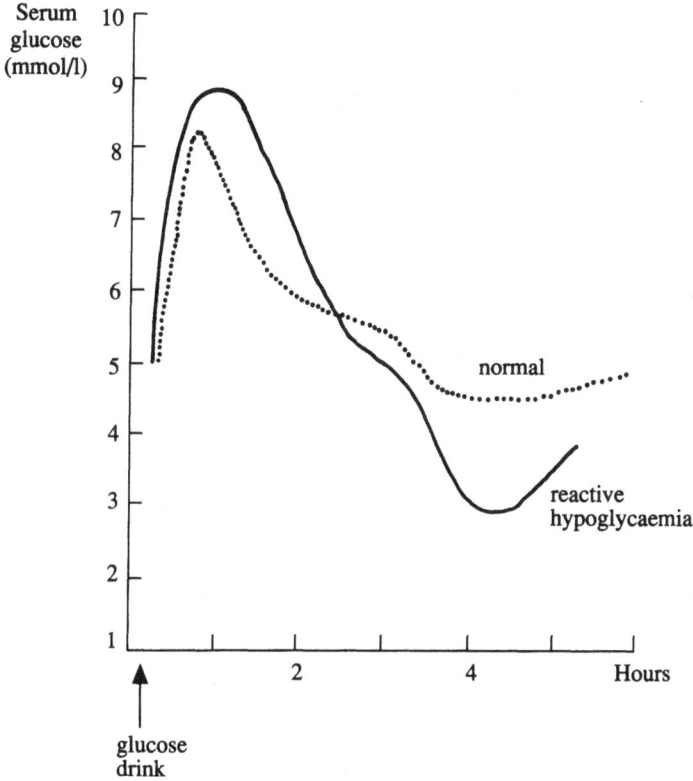

Fig. 24 The detection of reactive hypoglycaemia.

techniques to go into commercial production. Many companies soon dropped production of pig insulin altogether, and were horrified thereafter to see, in the medical
journals reports by patients of adverse reactions when using the human insulin.
Indeed, reports of sudden deaths in patients who had changed from porcine to
human insulin were received with alarm. The question as to whether human insulin
can increase the risk of fatal hypoglycaemia had to be answered.

Paradoxically, good control of blood glucose increases the risk of hypoglycaemia
since it lowers the concentration of glucose at which counterregulatory hormones
(growth hormone, cortisol) are released. There turned out to be no good evidence,

nonetheless, that human insulin adjusts this threshold differently from porcine insulin. An added factor is whether human insulin in some way alters a diabetic's **awareness** of his hypoglycaemia, in other words, the sweating and shaking, so that he is not aroused to find and ingest carbohydrate. The perception of these symptoms may be decreased by diabetic peripheral neuropathy, but no evidence has arisen to differentiate between the two sources of insulin in this respect either. So, you can expect to prescribe human recombinant insulin freely in the years ahead.

JUST KIDDING

A 40-year-old physiotherapist was seen by her general practitioner complaining of abdominal pain and loss of weight. As a precautionary procedure she was admitted to a surgical ward, and was noted to be clammy, sweaty and trembling; at one point she did lapse into coma. Blood was taken for examination and the most striking feature was a serum glucose of 1.8 mmol/l; this was soon raised by a dextrose infusion. A computerised tomography scan of the upper abdomen at this point revealed no abnormalities. However on being kept in for further observation she had fifteen hypoglycaemic episodes over the next few days. The insulin results began to come back — usually insulin is only measured once or twice a week even in the biggest and busiest laboratories — and were very high. The possible causes for the hypoglycaemia, at that point, were most of the items in the list above. However there seemed to be no infection, and tests of liver function were normal. More blood was taken and requests put in for a series of pituitary hormones measurements, but at that point an alert consultant phoned the laboratory and asked if they had any serum remaining from the previous insulin determinations. They did. He wanted them to analyse for C-peptide, which is the component of proinsulin split from insulin itself at the point of secretion. Endogenous insulin, from the patient's islets, is always accompanied by an equivalent amount of C-peptide. Administered insulin, human or porcine, does not contain it.

In this case the C-peptide values were very low. Surveillance was mounted on the patient and she was found to be injecting herself with commercial insulin from a syringe hidden in a box of paper tissues by the bedside. This is **factitious hypoglycaemia**. Most cases appear to occur in health-related professions, as in this instance. It is probably a variant of Munchhausen's syndrome, the compulsive relating of lies to gain medical attention.

ANOTHER GLUCOSE PROBLEM

A 29-year-old clerk complained of double vision on several occasions and later, his wife noticed that he seemed to be having fits while asleep. Referral to a neurologist and an extensive battery of laboratory and haematological tests, including a magnetic resonance imaging of the head, showed no abnormality. Thereafter his behaviour deteriorated, mainly in the direction of withdrawal and depression, and he had to give up working. Another set of tests including EEG showed no remarkable features. Recourse was then had to phenytoin (an anticonvulsant) and referral to a psychiatrist this time, who diagnosed a severe personality disorder. Further general non-specific complaints of illness and weakness led to a referral yet again, this time to a large well-equipped teaching hospital, where the professor of medicine reviewed all the possibilities:

(1) Drug intoxication
(2) Infection
(3) Renal failure
(4) Hepatic failure
(5) Hypoglycaemia
(6) Hypocalcaemia
(7) Porphyria
(8) Hypothyroidism
(9) Vitamin B deficiency
(10) Malignancy
(11) Systemic lupus erythematosus

All of these can yield a picture related to that seen in the patient, namely some sort of organic dementia. Nonetheless, most of them were extremely unlikely in view of the initial investigations. Ionised calcium, for instance, had been shown to be normal on several occasions, and kidney and liver function tests repeatedly showed that a disorder of these organs could be ruled out. B-vitamin (possibly thiamine or cobalamin) deficiency had not been seriously considered up to that point, nor had porphyria, nor lupus erythematosus. But they were kept in mind as the professor ordered blood chemistries every morning when the patient was fasting just before breakfast. The first day was unremarkable but the second day showed a serum glucose of 0.89 mmol/l. Over the next few days repeated determination of glucose alone in the blood from an indwelling catheter showed that there was episodic, acute hypoglycaemia. On laparotomy there was a tumour in the distal third of the pancreas. This was an insulinoma, a rare tumour, but even discounting its rarity, difficult to diagnose because of the non-specific nature of the symptoms — here confused with psychiatric disturbance.

HYPOGLYCAEMIA AND MALARIA

Erythrocytes containing mature parasites have a much enhanced glycolysis and therefore an enormous requirement for glucose. On top of that, fever enhances energy requirements in an infected host. The stress so imposed may not be cardinally important in adults, but as usual children are put at risk because of their comparatively small stores of liver glycogen and their greater brain to body ratio. In one instance, a girl was admitted with *Plasmodium falciparum* parasitaemia amd fever. Serum glucose was an alarming 0.52 mmol/l. Even after intravenous glucose administration, the concentration dropped to a staggeringly low 0.3 mmol/l and she died. In otherwise healthy individuals, the glucose deficit can be made up by gluconeogenesis using muscle and liver protein but in children in the tropics, there tends to be reduced capacity for this due to malnutrition and liver dysfunction. In any case, experts in the field recommend that close attention be paid to hypoglycaemia in children coming into hospital with infections, such as malaria and diarrhoea.

Further Reading

1. Gale EA. Hypoglycaemia and human insulin. *Lancet* ii 1264–1266, 1989.
2. Marks V. Diagnosis and differential diagnosis of hypoglycaemia. *Mayo Clinic Proceedings* **64** : 1558–1561, 1989.
3. White NJ, Miller KD, Marsh K, Berry CD, et al. Hypoglycaemia in African children with severe malaria. *Lancet* i : 708–711, 1987.

8a

Sudden Infant Death

The sudden infant death syndrome (SID) or "cot death" has been given considerable attention over the last decade and not surprisingly so, for it is a harrowing, if not devastating, experience for doctors and parents alike. It seems to happen to children aged between four weeks and one year, and as the name implies, they are found dead in the morning, quite suddenly and unexpectedly, having gone to sleep apparently well and healthy the night before. It now seems fairly certain that SID is a heterogeneous disorder, with some cases possibly attributable to abnormalities in respiratory control or to cardiac arrhythmias; others however display only non-specific indicators of illness at necroscopy. In one SID subgroup, fatty infiltration of the liver is observed, offering some resemblance to Reye's syndrome.

A Tangential Topic: Reye's Syndrome

This is an acute childhood illness, presenting with vomiting and coma, usually a few days after an apparent mild prodromal infection, which may be gastrointestinal or respiratory. Cerebral oedema and a fatty infiltration of the liver are salient features, but suspicion of Reye's will first be aroused by the signs of liver malfunction (marked rises in the transaminases and hyperammonaemia). Although the diagnosis of Reye's syndrome can be made on these clinical grounds, the pathogenesis remains unclear — it could be a result of a toxic agent or virus that causes a generalised mitochondrial dysfunction, probably in a genetically susceptible host. Aspirin administration has been implicated in some cases. Diagnosis in difficult situations can be helped by liver biopsy, which shows up the fatty vacuolation of the hepatocytes histologically, and the associated decrease in the activity of mitochondrial enzymes such as succinate dehydrogenase. On the whole though, it is difficult to recognise Reye's syndrome, and since it is often fatal, registers have been set up in many countries to collect notes of cases, and the physicians attached to these are experts who can proceed investigatively when suspicions arise.

In Reye's syndrome, the child is first observed to have lethargy, fits or coma, so is it part of an encehalopathic continuum which ranges from persistent drowsiness to the brain death in SID, where there is no chance to take blood specimens, biopsies or even a history, far less inatate treatment. We do not yet know. Nor do we know, in the case of Reye's syndrome in itself, how an apparently mild virus infection can lead to the serious liver derangements.

FATTY ACID OXIDATION DEFECTS

Some SID cases were however fairly definitely attributed to fatty acid oxidation defects. On autopsy the livers of these children had fatty infiltration of the liver, as in Reye's syndrome. Fresh tissues were handed over to investigative biochemists who assayed as many enzymes as possible related to fat metabolism. After numerous blind alleys they found that there was a deficiency of medium-chain acyl CoA dehydrogenase in the mitochondria. Here you again have to call up your hard-won knowledge of elementary biochemnistry. This enzyme is of course implicated in the β-oxidation pathway which (in conjunction with the citric acid cycle) yields carbon dioxide, water and energy in the form of ATP (Fig. 25). The fatty acids first have

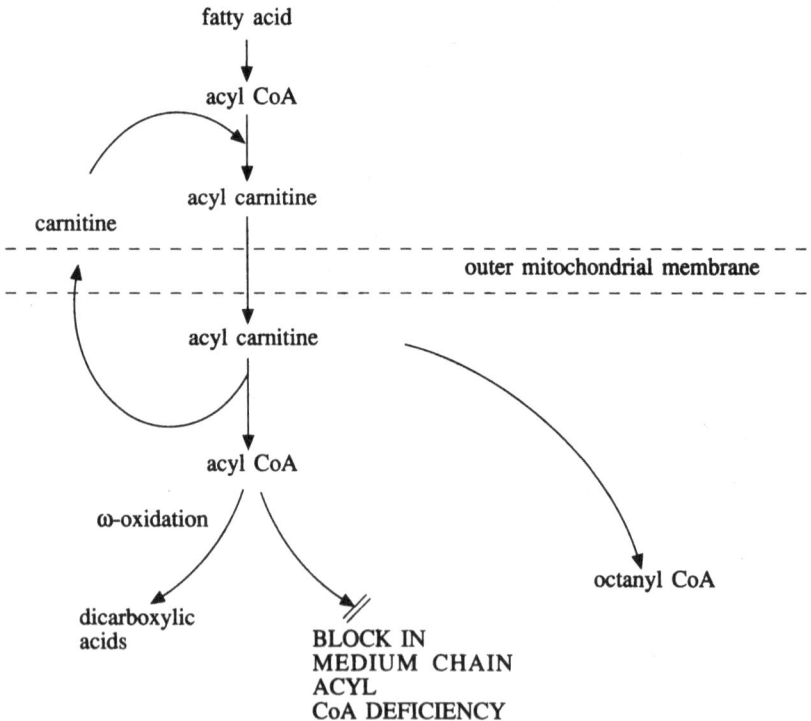

Fig. 25   The block in medium chain fatty acyl CoA deficiency.

This promotes the alternative pathways leading to dicarboxylic acids and octanoate.

to be "activated" by esterification with coenzyme A to form acyl CoA thioesters. A series of acyl CoA thiokinases are known to catalyse this reaction at the outer mitochondrial membrane, depending upon the chain length of the fatty acid concerned, i.e. short chain (2–3 carbon atoms), medium chain (4–12) or long chain (12–22). The activated fatty acids then cross the inner mitochondrial membrane where β-oxidation takes place. To facilitate this transport, the acyl CoA thioesters combine with carnitine, through the action of the enzyme acyl coenzyme A carnitine transferase. Having crossed the inner mitochondrial membrane, the acyl CoA thioesters are reformed by carnitine removal and they then undergo successive oxidative removal of acetyl CoA units from the carboxyl end. This whole reaction sequence is initiated by flavin adenine dinucleotide (FAD)-linked fatty acyl CoA dehydrogenases, again specific for short, medium and long chain substrates. The details of the rest of the β-oxidation pathway are not important in this context, for it is in the medium chain fatty acyl CoA dehydrogenase step that the primary defect associated with some cot deaths is thought to occur. The consequences are:

(1) Incomplete oxidation of fatty acids overall.
(2) Impaired ketone body production.
(3) Enhanced β-oxidation of medium chain fatty acids; oxidation occurs at the distal (non-carboxylic) end to replace β-oxidation. Thus large amounts of C6–C10 dicarboxylic acids and C6–C8 fatty acid conjugates are excreted in the urine of these patients. This represents a severe loss of the energy potentially available from the oxidation of the carbon chains.

CLINICAL IMPLICATIONS

Why do the children with this enzyme deficiency die so suddenly. The answer probably lies in item 2 above. Young children have precarious glycogen stores in their livers as compared to adults, supporting only a few hours of total fasting. Probably there has to be supplementation, in the early hours of the morning, with ketone bodies to preserve brain function. The situation will of course be aggravated if there has been poor feeding during the night before — parents for one reason or another might not be aware that this has been the case.

Some researchers have tried therapeutic addition of carnitine to the diet in infants deficient in medium chain fatty acid dehydrogenase, but who have survived, in this way hoping to facilitate the transport of the fatty acids across the mitochondrial membrane. Screening for high risk infants would be of considerable importance and it has been suggested that measuring medium chain fatty acid carnitine derivatives, such as octanoylcarnitine in the urine, may be useful. In addition, assay of the medium chain fatty acid dehydrogenase in skin fibroblasts may be tried.

DIAGNOSTIC ADVANCE

It was early assumed that the dehydrogenase deficiency is probably genetic — for a start, families with more than one cot death were often documented. Confirmation of this was strikingly obtained by workers in North Carolina (Ref. 3 below) who retrieved the paraffin sections of two sisters who had died of unknown causes. (Some liver tissue had been removed at autopsy for histology, but no abnormality had been found.) The DNA from the sections was prepared and portions of it corresponding to an amino acid sequence of the medium chain acyl dehydrogenase were amplified by PRC (see Chap. 3a). The same was done on leukocytic DNA from a newborn sister in the same family, as well as from the parents and from one more, apparently normal, sister. This amplified DNA was treated with a restriction endonuclease which cuts it in two if it is normal, but leaves it intact if there is an adenine to guanine mutation (previously well characterised.) The existence of these fragments is of course discovered by looking at bands on polyacrylamide gel after electrophoresis. The results can be summarised:

newborn	normal sister	father	mother	deceased sister 1	deceased sister 2
one band	*two bands*	*two bands*	*two bands*	*one band*	*one band*

Therefore both parents are probably heterozygotic for the mutation in the dehydrogenase and the neonate is affected; she has to be watched carefully, given supplemental carnitine, and not left for long periods overnight without nourishment.

Comment

Other enzyme deficiencies may be found in SID children. But before that, here is a conundrum. Why is SID rare in the tropics? You might hypothesise that hypothermia plays a part in many cases in northern climes, and this has been suggested too. But a more likely explanation lies in the social behaviour of families in the East and West. In the latter, parents like to get their children to bed fairly early, both because this is thought to be good for them, in terms of rest, and because they (the parents) would like an uninterrupted and peaceful evening. In the tropics even quite young children are allowed to run around the house until very late, until they themselves feel tired, and they probably have a high carbohydrate (rice) snack before they do eventually drop off. Relatively then, the Western children are exposed to a much longer period of potential hypoglycaemia. If there is some other factor compromising energy supply, such as medium chain fatty acyl CoA deficiency, the difference may well be crucial.

Further Reading

1. Anon. Sudden infant death and inherited disorders of fat oxidation. *Lancet* **ii** : 1073, 1986.
2. Dezateux CA, Dinwiddie R, Helms P and Mathew DJ. Recognition and early management of Reye's syndrome. *Arch Dis Childhood.* **63** : 647–651, 1986.
3. Ding JH, Roe CR, Iafolla AK and Chen YT. Medium chain acyl CoA dehydrogenase deficiency and sudden infant death. *N Eng J Med* **325** : 61, 1991.

8b

In Praise of Fish Oil

The Eskimos had always presented something of a metabolic puzzle to those interested enough to study them, for example, where did they obtain their vitamin C, which largely comes from fresh fruits and vegetables in diets throughout the rest of the world? (It turned out that they eat the mossy contents of the stomachs of the caribou; also, it could be that seal and whale meat — especially if uncooked, the word "eskimo" meaning someone who eats raw flesh — contains enough of the vitamin to get them by.) In addition, in the late 1970s it became apparent that the Eskimos of north-west Greenland had a very low incidence of coronary heart disease, despite a diet laden with highly saturated and cholesterol-laden seal, polar bear and walrus fat. But they also ate a large amount of fish and nutritionists wondered if the apparent protection of the heart was associated with a high fish consumption. A similar relationship was also implied from studies in Japan and in other communities largely favouring fish consumption. Dutch researchers had also described an inverse relationship between fish consumption and coronary artery disease, indeed they found mortality from this to be decreased by more than 50% in subjects who ate at least 30g of fish a day in their diet, as compared to non- or minimal-fish eaters. Although association does not mean causality, there was enough evidence to warrant further investigation of what might be the protective component of fish.

After casting around a bit, the investigators decided that polyunsaturated fatty acids were likely to be the protective factors. Fish, because they acquire them in the food chain from marine phytoplankton, are rich in the long chain n–3 polyunsaturated fatty acids, namely eicosapentaenoic acid (C20:5 n–3) and docosahexaenoic acid (C22:6 n–3). These confusing numbers and designations need some explanation. We have to describe an unsaturated fatty acid by the total number of carbon atoms and the distribution of the double bonds. A simple member of the series is oleic acid which has eighteen carbon atoms and one double bond between positions 9 and 10, which by convention are counted from the carboxyl group. It can readily be identified as C18:1 in that light. But an alternative nomenclature defines the double bonds in terms of their distance from the non-carboxyl, or omega end of the molecule. Thus oleic acid could be described as C18:1 ω–9 or alternatively C18:1 n–9. For some reason it is this last nomenclature which has stuck, especially in the medical literature. Thus eicosapentaenoic acid or C20:5 n–3 has 20 carbons and 5 double bonds, the "first" of which is 3 carbons from the non-carboxyl end. It is understood that in polyunsaturated fatty acids the other double bonds are always three carbons distant from each other. To make it, we hope, even more clear, the formula for eicosapentaenoic would look like this when written out in full.

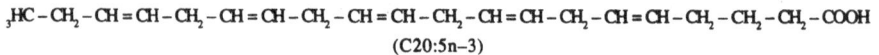

$_3$HC – CH$_2$ – CH = CH – CH$_2$ – CH = CH – CH$_2$ – CH = CH – CH$_2$ – CH = CH – CH$_2$ – CH = CH – CH$_2$ – CH$_2$ – CH$_2$ – COOH

(C20:5n–3)

These unsaturated fatty acids may be as important for fish as they are for humans, for unlike their more saturated homologues they have very low melting points and so do not solidify and make movement impossible in cold Arctic seas. Even so, there is a wide variation among edible fish — mackerel for example has about 2.5 g/100g of n–3 fatty acids, canned sardines about 1.7 and less oily fish like cod only 0.2.

Humans do not have the ability to synthesise fatty acids with double bonds that are more distal than the 9th carbon, in this convention the 1st carbon being the carboxyl bearing one. Thus linoleic acid (C18:2 n–6) the main polyunsaturated fatty acid of corn oil, for example, cannot be synthesised by humans and must therefore be obtained from the diet — in other words it is an essential fatty acid. It can however be converted to arachidonic acid (C20:4 n–6) by elongation by two carbon atoms then desaturation to form two extra double bonds. Arachidonic acid is an important physiological compound as it is the precursor of the eicosanoids, i.e oxygenated products of 20-carbon polyunsaturated fatty acids which consist of the leukotrienes derived from lipoxygenase pathways and also prostaglandins and thromboxanes formed from the cyclooxygenase pathways (Fig. 26)

Another essential fatty acid, α-linolenic acid (C18:3 n–3) is found in soybean and rape-seed oils. However the amount of eicosapentaenoic acid or docosa hexaenoic acid which can be produced from it in humans is probably small and thus fish oils constitute the main source of these fatty acids.

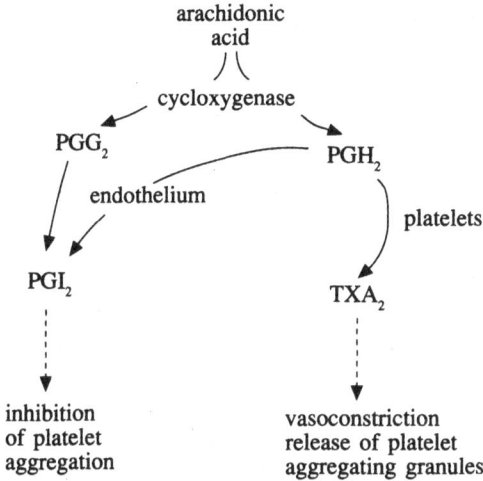

arachidonic
acid

cycloxygenase

PGG_2

PGH_2

endothelium

platelets

PGI_2

TXA_2

inhibition
of platelet
aggregation

vasoconstriction
release of platelet
aggregating granules

PGG_2, PGH_2 = endoperoxide ($- C \overset{O}{——} C -$) intermediates

PGI_2 = prostacyclin

TXA_2 = thromboxane A

Fig. 26 Summary of arachidonic acid metabolism.

Dietary (fish oil) n–3 polyunsaturates, by means of their oxidised intermediates, may in some way tip the balance in favour of the left hand branch of this sequence.

How do these n–3 compounds exert a cardioprotective action? Referring back to the Eskimo studies, it was observed that total cholesterol and low density lipoprotein (LDL) were lower in Eskimos than in control populations eating less fish. Although subsequent trials with other populations fed either fish oils or the pure n–3 fatty acids have not been entirely uniform in their outcomes (such trials never are), the hypolipidaemic effect has been more or less confirmed. In one striking experiment; either a fish oil or a normal diet was fed to chickens, then the egg yolks from these chickens were fed to human vounteers; only the yolks from the chickens on the normal diets raised the serum cholesterol. The effect of the n–3 fatty acids has been attributed to the lowering of very low density lipoproteins (VLDL) which are the precursors of LDL. The mechanism of this may be that n–3 fatty acids increase VLDL removal from the circulation and also decrease triglyceride synthesis by the liver.

A second mode of action might be as a modulator of inflammation. The n–3 fatty acids can serve as substrates for lipoxygenase activity, producing leukotrienes, which are involved in inflammatory processes such as chemoattraction. The evidence is that they make the neutrophils, monocytes and macrophages less chemotactic and this might be important in the developing atheroma, which is infiltrated by the lipid laden cells, called foam cells which are recruited by an infammation-like sequence of events.

Then again, other important actions of n–3 fatty acids, principally eicosopentaenoic and docosahexaenoic acids, concern haemostasis and the vascular system. They can compete with arachidonic acid for substitution into membrane phospholipids and also competitively inhibit the conversion of arachidonic acid, in platelets, to thromboxane A2, a very potent platelet aggregating agent and vasoconstrictor. On the other hand in endothelia the n–3 acids probably inhibit the conversion of arachidonic acid to prostaglandin I2 (prostacyclin) which competes with thromboxane 2A, since it is vasodilatory and inhibitory of platelet aggregation and adhesion to blood vessel walls. Somehow or other, the n–3 polyunsaturates tip the balance in favour of the endothelium against the platelets; this is important because the latter can release platelet derived growth factor, which is capable of aiding the proliferation of smooth muscle cells within the intima of damaged blood vessels, further amplifying atheroma formation.

Thus the n–3 fatty acids found in fish oils have a number of pharmacological actions of particular relevance to thrombotic and inflammatory situations. They have been rendered into capsules by the pharmaceutical companies and are undergoing trials, not only on the topics mentioned above, but on a whole range of other pathologies. For example, they may also have a role in reducing the "leakage" of albumin into the urine of insulin dependent diabetics (so-called microalbuminuria, see Chap. 2a) possibly by reducing the permeability of the glomerular capillaries. It seems also to be relatively well established that the n–3 fatty acids can lower blood pressure, but whether or not this is due to altered production of prostaglandins remains to be settled.

Comment

One can learn a lot about the pathophysiology and biochemistry of atherosclerosis and vascular disease from reading around the subject of fish oils. In practical terms though, caution is necessary as high-dose cod liver oil, if that is used as the source, contains large quantities of the potentially toxic fat soluble vitamins A and D, as well as causing bleeding problems and bruising in some individuals.

Further Reading

1. Nordoy A. Fish oils in clinical medicine. *J Intern Med* **225** : 145–146, 1989.
2. Kinsella JE, Lokesh B and Stone RA. Dietary n–3 polyunsaturated fatty acids and amelioration of cardiovascular disease: possible mechanisms. *Am J Clin Nutr* **52** : 1–28, 1990.

9a
Nitrogen Disposal Problems

The paediatrician is often confronted with a severe problem in the infant who is just generally ill but cannot easily be ascribed any diagnosis. Typically, it may be "failure to thrive" with one or more of a number of other manifestations such as:
(1) Convulsions
(2) Hypotonia or flaccidity of the muscles
(3) Persistent vomiting
(4) Drowsiness
(5) One, some or all of — lactic acidosis, hypoglycaemia, hyperammonaemia, ketosis

An inborn error of metabolism is suspected, but there are about one thousand different possibilities. Nonetheless, mentally or on paper, there will be a flow chart to narrow down the options. Perhaps consideration of the commonest inherited diseases in the country and/or the ethnic group involved will help. Certainly renal, cardiac and infectious diseases will have been excluded by this time, using routine laboratory tests, so that a more specialised strategy is required to pinpoint the precise defect.

A SPECIFIC PRESENTATION

In one such case, the child, a boy (it is of paramount importance, of course, to note and remember the sex, for the condition may turn out to be sex-linked) was born two months before being brought back to hospital. Ammonia, lactic acid and bilirubin were all high but there was no hypoglycaemia or ketosis. There is a strong indication here of some liver defect, but because of the normoglycaemia, glycogen storage disease is unlikely. In any case, the first step is to try to obtain some blood for investigation, then adopt emergency measures to rid the body of the very toxic ammonia. In this case, peritoneal dialysis was first instituted; in this manoeuvre fluid is infused into the abdominal cavity and the toxins from the thoracic cavity diffuse into it through the peritoneum and can thereby be drained out through an exit line. A second emergency step was to feed benzoic acid solution, the rationale for which is as follows: the acid combines readily with glycine to give the easily diffusible and therefore excretable hippuric acid. Glycine itself is readily formed from glyoxylate when there is an excess of ammonia in the liver. An artificial conduit for the removal of nitrogen is thus created:

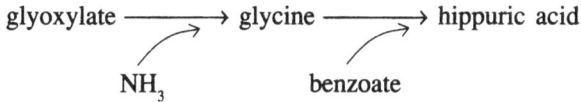

$$\text{glyoxylate} \xrightarrow[\quad\nearrow\quad]{} \text{glycine} \xrightarrow[\quad\nearrow\quad]{} \text{hippuric acid}$$
$$\qquad\quad NH_3 \qquad\qquad\quad \text{benzoate}$$

With these maintenance steps taken, the paediatricians in this case were free to consider possible investigations of the baseline blood. Hyperammonaemia, which is the most critical abnormality in the first instance, may have many causes, thus:

(1) Carnitine deficiency
(2) Reye's syndrome
(3) Valproic acid administration (an antiepileptic drug)
(4) Organic acidurias
(5) Urea cycle defects — which can be due to at least five enzyme deficiencies — carbamyl phosphate synthetase, ornithine transcarbamylase, argininosuccinate synthetase, argininosuccinase, arginase

In the case we are documenting here, some of these could be eliminated. Valproate, which has an amino group releasing ammonia on metabolism, had not been given. A supplementation of carnitine failed to reduce the hyperammonaemia (carnitine deficit causes hyperammonaemia by blocking fatty acid oxidation and causing massive amino acid catabolism). Reye's syndrome (see further about this disease in Chap. 8a) perhaps could not be ruled out immediately but was unlikely due to the absence of convulsions and the relatively normal serum transaminases. Hyperammonaemia in organic acidurias is a secondary phenomenon and equally could not be ruled out at an early stage; however the baby was unlikely to have maple syrup urine disease — a defect in the metabolism of the branched chain amino acids — which is usually fatal very early in infancy.

An amino acid chromatogram was done as rapidly as possible. Even with today's technology this sort of test generally involves an overnight delay at the minumum, so there was an anxious period of waiting for the result, which was as in Fig. 27. A normal, healthy child's serum amino acids are shown for comparison. You will see that the patterns are quite complex. The laboratory will help you in the interpretation, but you know from elementary biochemistry that whereas there are twenty or so amino acids in protein hydrolysates, there are more than that in the serum, some of them with physiological functions of their own, such as glutamine (transporting substrate from the muscles to the liver) and taurine (a constituent of the bile salts). In the patient, glutamine, alanine and glycine all seem to be high. These are all physiological sinks for ammonia:

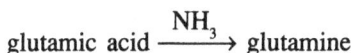

$$\text{glutamic acid} \xrightarrow{NH_3} \text{glutamine}$$

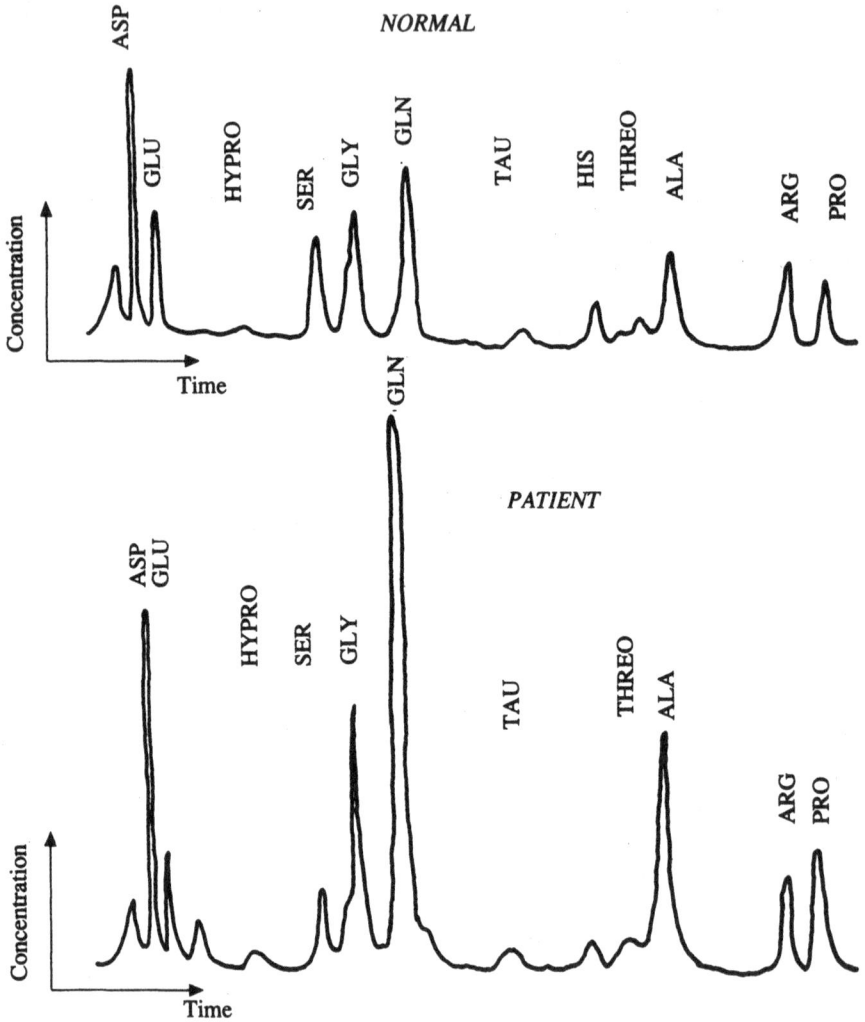

ASP = aspartic acid; GLU = glutamic acid; HYPRO = hydroxyproline;
SER = serine; TAU = taurine; THREO = threonine;
ARG = arginine; PRO = proline; HIS = histidine.

Fig. 27 Serum amino acid patterns.

These sequences of peaks represent the first parts of the two elution patterns; the child with the suspected inherited disorder has a greatly enhanced glutamine (GLN) peak and to some extent glycine (GLY) and alanine (ALA) are also enhanced. It is normal for there to be small unidentifiable peaks, especially in pathological samples.

$$\text{pyruvate} \xrightarrow{\text{NH}_3} \text{alanine}$$

$$\text{glyoxylate} \xrightarrow{\text{NH}_3} \text{glycine}$$

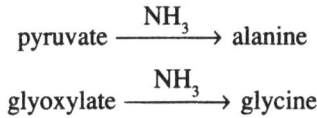

(A fourth possible sink, asparagine, which is formed from aspartic acid and ammonia, is not well separated from glycine in the two chromatograms.) The initial impression is that all the substrates which can become loaded with excess nitrogen, have become so, because there is no outlet for nitrogen as urea, in other words, there is a urea cycle disorder. None of the urea cycle amino acids, such as argininosuccinate, arginine or citrulline, is high, suggesting that the cycle does not even get started — so this must be ornithine transcarbamylase or carbamyl phosphate synthetase deficiency. One further investigation is going to clinch this case — the presence or absence of large amounts of orotic acid in the urine, and the reason for this can be seen by referring to Fig. 28. Were the defect carbamyl phosphate synthetase deficiency, there would be no substrate for orotic acid synthesis; were it ornithine transcarbamylase deficiency, then orotic acid will act as another sink for removal of the build-up of excess nitrogen. Orotic acid is easily measured, and there turned out to be large amounts of it in the urine of the baby, who was suffering from ornithine transcarbamylase deficiency. Ornithine itself is not usually high in this disease — as one can work out from the diagram, it is not produced at all.

The condition is an X-linked dominant one. It is usually highly lethal in boys, and the child described here survived longer than might have been expected. There are however intermediate, less severe forms in which some urea appears to be synthesised. It is less severe in girls due to lyonisation — this is the process by which one of the two X-chromosomes in each cell of the normal female becomes genetically inactive at an early stage of embryogenesis. It is a random matter whether the inactivated chromosome comes from the father or the mother and so if a girl inherits an X-linked mutation from one parent its effect is halved.

The treatment for ornithine transcarbamylase deficiency is protein restriction. The cause of the lactic acidosis in this particular case remained obscure — perhaps the hyperammonaemia was high enough to make the child alkalotic and so depress the respiratory centre, in a physiological response designed to retain carbonic acid.

Comment

In the case recounted above, the child gradually deteriorated and treatment was withdrawn shortly before he passed away. Everybody knows that autopsies are often done after death but few are aware that the biochemistry laboratory may be at work on the body fluids of a child who has died of an undiagnosed condition long after the unfortunate loss; this of course is to try to establish the exact illness in the interests of advice to the parents before or during any future pregnancy. Nowadays

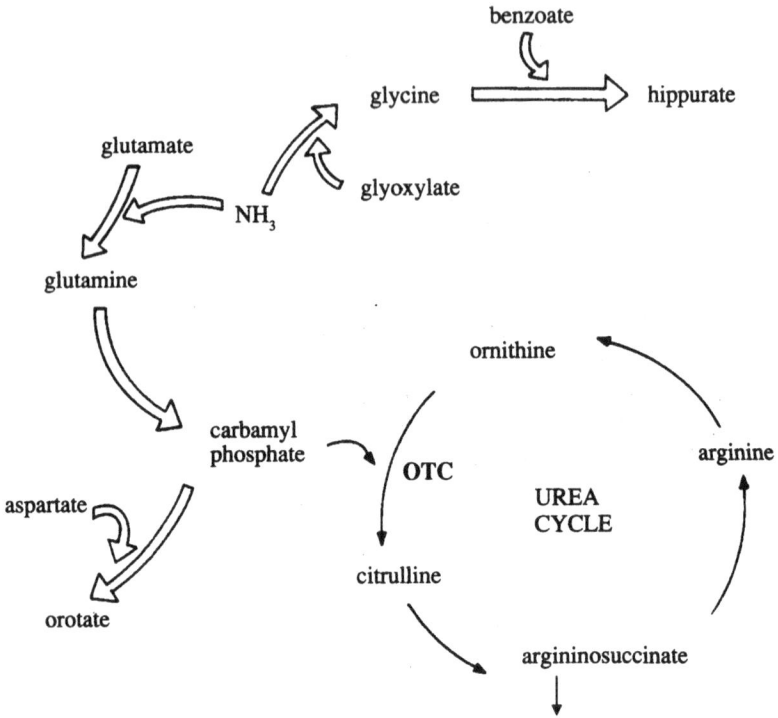

Fig. 28   Patterns of nitrogen disposal in ornithine transcarbamylase (OTC) deficiency.

With the entry of NH_3 into the urea cycle blocked by lack of the enzyme, it is taken up by other acceptors as shown by the thickened arrows. Benzoate can be administered to trap the glycine as hippurate which is excreted in the urine. (Here for brevity all the acids are expressed as the anion form, for example "orotate" instead of "orotic acid".)

one would certainly wish to store some cellular material since for many inherited diseases DNA probes are available to pinpoint the defect; as they become more informative they can be used in conjunction with genomic DNA which has been banked for many years beforehand, and will allow the tracking of the mutation in families. There are probes for ornithine transcarbamylase deficiency already, but in the case, cited the diagnosis was arrived at without recourse to them; the aim was to save the child, and the exact mutation a matter of peripheral interest to the paediatricians under the circumstances.

In adults, the determination of blood ammonia is important in liver failure. Because of the resulting coma, the manifestation is known as hepatic encephalopathy — almost all the clinical symptoms of hyperammonaemia, in adults and children, are connected with the central nervous system.

Further Reading

1. Bachman C. Diagnosis of urea cycle disorders. *Recent Advances in Inborn Errors of Metabolism* **38** : 233–241, 1987.
2. Harkness RA. Clinical biochemistry of the neonatal period. *J Clin Pathol* **40** : 1128–1144, 1987.
3. Applegarth DA, Dimmick JE and Toone JR. Laboratory detection of metabolic disease. *Pediatr Clin N Am* **36** : 49–66, 1989.

9b

NO Relaxing with Arginine

Nitric oxide was discovered by Priestley about two hundred years ago. Its simple formula, NO conceals some rather important properties. It is better written as $\bullet N = O$ meaning that it is a free radical, the dot representing an unpaired electron and making it highly chemically reactive, so much so that it came as a surprise to find it could be synthesised by mammalian cells at all. In industry it can be described as a toxic gas. Indeed on the face of it its synthesis seems further to be highly undesirable in that it is one of the constituents of tobacco smoke and polluted air. Once in the lungs, it can go on to react with hydrogen peroxide generated from pulmonary macrophages and neutrophils to produce the highly obnoxious hydroxyl free radical.

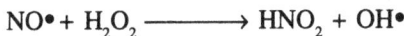

$$NO\bullet + H_2O_2 \longrightarrow HNO_2 + OH\bullet$$

It seemed until recently, then, a chemical much to be avoided by intact cells.

It had long been known that acetylcholine can relax isolated blood vessels as long as the endothelium — the single layer of cells so important in maintaining the liquidity and integrity of the blood — is present. Paradoxically, however, acetylcholine is a constrictor agonist when blood vessels are studied in vitro in tissue baths, suggesting that in vivo this agent releases some secondary factor which acts rapidly and locally, undisturbed by the artefactual conditions of the experiment itself. Consequently, a humoral factor was postulated and named endothelium-dependent relaxing factor (EDRF). It was shown not to be prostacyclin, a recognised potent endothelial derived vasodilator (Chap. 8b) as it could still express its action in the presence of indomethacin, a drug known to interfere with prostacyclin production by inhibiting cyclooxygenase pathways. Work by Salvador Moncada has identified EDRF as being chemically related to, or identical with, NO. Further, he has demonstrated that it is a product of the amino acid L-arginine, but not the D-arginine isomer; this of course indicates that it a product of enzymic action. The exact details of the process are still the centre of extensive research but there is involvement of an NO synthetase, a cytosolic NADPH-dependent enzyme which may exist as different isoenzymes in different tissues. Also, preliminary reports suggest that tetrahydrobiopterin is a cofactor for L-arginine oxidation and that an initial reaction product is L-hydroxylarginine. The L-arginine analogue N-monomethyl-L-arginine (L-NMMA), can inhibit L-arginine generation of NO, emphasising again the stereospecificity of the reaction.

A detailed insight into these pathways is of potential therapeutic importance in the context of developing drugs with vasodilating properties. Synthetic nitrovasodilators such as the anti-anginal agent glyceryl trinitrate, whose used was based on quite empirical observations, can now be rationalised as NO producers in certain tissues.

NO ACTION

NO has a number of actions and functions:
(1) It is able to relax arterioles, arteries and veins.
(2) It can inhibit platelet aggregation induced by thrombin, collagen, ADP and platelet activating factor.
(3) It can inhibit platelet adhesion to endothelial cells.
(4) It acts as a neurotransmitter, e.g. in the stomach, to relax its smooth muscle on intake of food (receptive relaxation).

Its non-neurotransmitter actions are mediated through its stimulation of intracellular guanylate cyclase, which results in increases in intracellular cyclic GMP; this enzyme is analogous to adenylate cyclase that produces cyclic AMP, another intracellular messenger molecule. The cyclic GMP modulates intracellular calcium levels resulting in relaxation of smooth muscle in synergy with the analogous intracellular secondary "messenger", cyclic AMP. The mechanism of action of NO on platelets is probably similar.

NO has a short half-life — possibly only seconds — which suggests that it may have a relatively localised site of action on the smooth muscle cells and platelets subsequent to its synthesis by endothelium. In any event it is speedily oxidised in the presence of oxygen to form NO_2 and NO_3. Superoxide anions (O_2^-) which can be synthesised by endothelial cells, also inactivates NO as does binding to haemoglobin and haptoglobin complexes within the plasma.

Other vasodilators can interact with NO by activating membrane-associated adenylate cyclase and, as mentioned above, increasing intracellular cyclic AMP to lower intracellular calcium and thus relax smooth muscle. Such vasodilating agents include prostacyclin and β-adrenergic agonists like adrenaline — NO would therefore be expected to be important in the synergy of vascular responses.

The actions of NO upon vasoactivity and platelet function are also important in pathological situations. It is known that in atherosclerosis there is an impairment in vascular relaxation, and it has been proposed that low density lipoproteins, particularly if oxidised, can reduce NO production by endothelial cells. Another suggestion is that the vasospasm of cerebral vessels following a subarachnoid haemorrhage may be in part a result of the inactivation of NO by haemoglobin. Whether or not the thickening of the intimal layer of atheromatous blood vessels results in impaired diffusion of NO from the endothelium to the smooth muscle and thus contributes to reduced vasodilatation is a question which will be answered in due course.

The roles of NO in other cells and tissues are also of considerable interest. White cells appear to have the capacity to release NO, and cytokines such as interferon-γ, interleukin-1 and tumour necrosis factor may have the ability to facilitate NO release from endothelial cells. The liver may also be able to synthesise NO as a protection against sepsis.

A THERAPEUTIC ROLE FOR ARGININE

Recently arginine has been perfused into the coronary vessels of patients with hypercholesterolaemia, in an attempt to improve coronary flow, on the basis that it had previously been shown to be a rate limiting factor in the production of EDRF. The conclusion was that the impaired coronary microcirculation in such subjects can indeed be restored by the short term administration of the amino acid as a precusor of the effector substance.

Arginine is also a potent secretagogue, in that it enhances the activity of many endocrine glands; this is used in the detection of growth hormone deficiency, for infusion of it into patients fails to provoke the normal rise of hormone in the serum.

Further Reading

1. Griffith T and Randall M. Nitric oxide comes of age. *Lancet* **ii** : 875–876, 1989.

2. Palmer RJM Ashton DS and Moncado S. Vascular endothelial cells synthesise nitric oxide from L-arginine. *Nature* **333** : 875–876, 1989.
3. Botting R and Vane JR. Mediators and anti-thrombotic properties of the vascular endothelium. *Ann Med* **21** : 31–38, 1989.
4. Editorial. Nitric oxide in the clinical arena. *Lancet* **ii** : 1560–1563, 1991.

9c

Tyrosine, Multiple Endocrine Neoplasia, and the Elephant Man

The term phaeochromocytoma was first coined in 1912 by Pick, to characterise a tumour of chromaffin cells. He used this terminology because microscopic sections of the tumour, when stained with chromium salts, gave a typical pattern of catecholamine storage granules. This tumour is of clinical significance as one of the endocrine causes of hypertension, due to the release of vasopressive biogenic amines. Indeed, although phaeochromocytomas are present in only about five in one hundred thousand people (which we could consider rare), they do constitute the reason for about five in every thousand cases of hypertension. A further unusual feature of this tumour is its familial tendency, with about 10% of sufferers having a positive family history and in whom there is an increased propensity for bilateral tumours, that is, both the medullas of the adrenal glands are affected. However, the adrenal is not the only site of this tumour — it can develop at any anatomical site where primitive sympathetic nerve cells or chromaffin cells remain, such as the urinary bladder wall or the para-aortic bodies.

Another curious fact is that phaeochromocytomas are associated with other diseases, notably neurofibromatosis (also called von Recklinghausen's disease, famous since the "Elephant Man" in the film — who may have been a sufferer from it) and also as one of the possible features of the multiple endocrine neoplasia type 2 syndrome (MEN 2) or Sipple's syndrome. This latter has been the focus of some recent biochemical and genetic research as an example of an inherited cancer, apparently autosomal dominant. In the MEN 2 syndrome, tumours of the thyroid C cells or calcitonin producing cells (so-called medullary thyroid carcinoma) are found in association with phaeochromocytomas. This is also an association with hyperparathyroidism. Furthermore, there are complexities as the syndrome manifests heterogeneity of expression, with one variant MEN 2B associated with a more aggressive nature of tumour growth with an earlier onset in life, and also skeletal abnormalities. Its gene has been localised to chromosome 10. For completeness, we note here that the type 1 syndrome, also known as Werner's syndrome, has another pattern of endocirne tumour association, namely pituitary adenomas, pancreatic islet cell tumours (insulinomas, gastrinomas and glucagonomas) and primary hyperparathyroidism.

What is the biochemical contribution in this context, for clinical examination is often not very helpful, as symptoms can be non-specific, with no obvious pathognomonic features? Patients often complain of sweating, palpitations and "funny turns", and they can have detectable hypertension and glycosuria — these are all typical results of an excess of the sympathomimetic amines, but can be consequences in whole or in part of many other diseases. The result is, as one famous study of postmortems over a fifty-year period in the United States demonstrated, most phaeochromocytomas are missed. The biochemical tests which are useful can best be understood by a refresher diagram such as Fig. 29, illustrating catecholamine metabolism. The laboratory, then, will be prepared to measure:

(1) Plasma or urine adrenaline and noradrenaline — they would theoretically be expected to be raised in patients with phaeochromocytomas. However, the secretion from the tumour tends to be sporadic, and so a surge into plasma can easily be missed. A twenty-four hour urine is a better specimen, but even then can be non-informative during a quiescent period. Plasma sampling comes into its own when you are sure that there is a tumour in the medulla but wish to know whether it is on the right or left — in that case, a catheter can be introduced into the inferior vena cava to find out. Then the surgical operation for removal is easier.

(2) Metanephrines (normetadrenaline and metadrenaline) which are a product of the catalytic action of the enzyme catechol-O-methyl transferase. They are excreted in the urine and can also be routinely measured, albeit with some difficulty.

(3) 4-hydroxy-3-methoxy-mandelic acid (HMMA) often called vanillylmandelic acid (VMA) which is the further metabolic products of the metanephrines due initially to the activity of the enzyme monoamine oxidase (MAO) and then another more obscure oxidation process involving an acid and aldehyde. VMA is evidently the ultimate sink for all the active substances and

metabolites (although there are other, minor pathways).
How does this all work in practice?

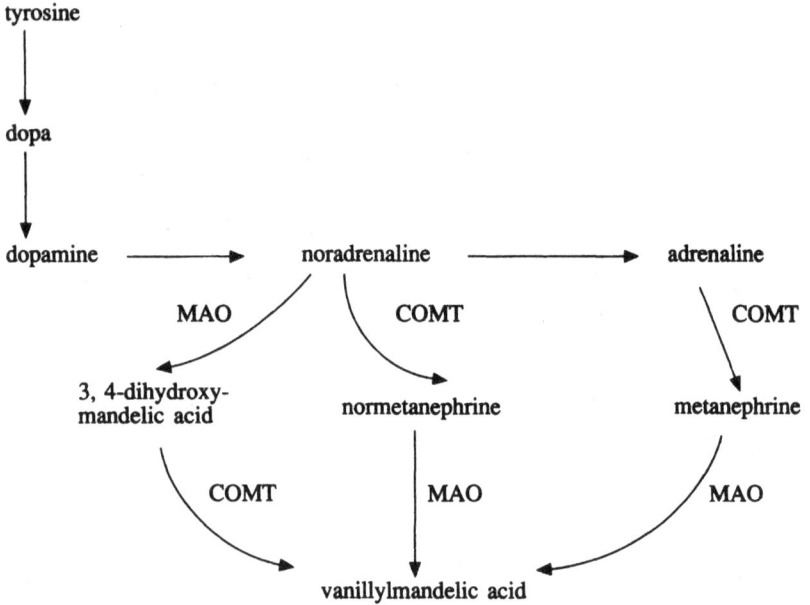

MAO = monamine oxidase
COMT = catechol-O-methyl transferase

Fig. 29 Summary of catecholamine metabolism.

Vanillylmandelic acid (VMA) is alternatively known as 4-hydroxy-3-methylmandelic acid (HMMA). If one is using the terms adrenaline and noradrenaline rather than epinephrine and norepinephrine it would certainly be more logical to call their products metadrenaline and normetadrenaline respectively, but the more familiar terms for the "mets" are given in the diagram.

TAKING TO THE (URINE) BOTTLE

A 43-year-old insurance clerk saw his general practitioner because he felt periodically unwell, complaining of headaches, dizziness, shaking and sweatiness. The doctor noted a thin, anxious looking individual who confessed to feeling inadequte about his work and social life and to be taking large amounts of vitamins and health foods in response to advertisements in a magazine he subscribed to. The physical examination was unremarkable, the blood pressure on that occasion being 140/95. The doctor took some blood for a few tests and asked the patient to try to come and see him or one of his colleagues in the practice during one of the periods of dizziness, if such should recur. The initial results were:

sodium	140	mmol/l	(reference interval, 135–150)
potassium	4.5	mmol/l	(3.5–5)
urea	5.6	mmol/l	(3.2–7.5)
creatinine	90	μmol/l	(70–130)
glucose (random)	9.7	mmol/l	(4–7.8)

The rather high glucose suggested that a glucose tolerance test should be performed, and an appointment was made at the clinical chemistry department of the local hospital. The chemical pathologist followed through the blood glucose determinations over the two hours, but they were not diagnostic of diabetes. (The patient had of course come fasting, and the basal glucose concentration was 6.9 mmol/l, just slightly higher than normal.) Looking at the notes, he phoned up the general practitioner and suggested that the patient be given a bottle for a twenty-four hour specimen of urine, the collection to start as soon as the feelings of unease commenced, and this was agreed upon. In the urine, sent ten days later, the laboratory found the following:

metanephrines	3500	nmol/day	(reference interval 250–1700)
HMMA (VMA)	85	μmol/day	(1.5–39)

A diagnosis of phaeochromocytoma then seemed very probable; the doctor managed to record a very high blood pressure (184/120) during one of the attacks and then arranged for nuclear magnetic resonance imaging, which had just become available at the nearest university medical centre. This revealed a substantial left-sided adrenal phaeochromocytoma, which was successfully removed at operation, with a complete recovery of the patient who subsequently became normotensive and whose fasting blood glucose returned to normal.

Phaeochromocytoma is an example of a tumour secreting, in an episodic manner, the natural products of the untransformed cells, which can be detected and quantitated, usually after some persistent investigation. The catecholamines, metanephrines and HMMA/VMA collectively are of course a special type of tumour marker (cf Chap. 1c)

Further Reading

1. Coulson RC and Brown MJ. Catecholamine measurements in phaeochromocytoma. *Ann Clin Biochem* **19** : 346–404, 1982.
2. Bone HG. Diagnosis of the multiglandular endocrine neoplasias. *Clin Chem* **36** : 711–717, 1990.

10a

Starvation: Biochemistry and the Melting of Solid Flesh

About a hundred years ago, the Polish banker Conrad Bloch predicted that thenceforth famine would be the main instrument of warfare, and he has been proved only too right. In this century, war has made starvation the commonest of the severe pathological experiences of mankind (unless the "accolade" has to be handed to malaria), but in addition, as a medical problem it extends to a number of settings:
  (1) Inanition in surgical patients
  (2) Cachexia of cancer
  (3) Anorexia and bulimia nervosa
  (4) Religious and political fasting
  (5) Therapeutic starvation
  In none of these situations is the mere availability of food remedial, and even in the refeeding of refugees care is required, as explained below.

METABOLIC COURSE OF STARVATION

Variations in the metabolic pattern of starvation from whatever cause are due to differences in the starting point, that is the body composition of the individual concerned. Take however a 60 kg man about to start on a total fast. He would be a fairly small individual, just under ten stones by the old means of reckoning, perhaps more typical of the tropics, and he maintains about the quantities of energy stores shown in Table 3. Note that the nutrients are available in very unequal quantities, and that they also yield different amounts of energy. However on the first day of the fast, there is a total depletion of liver glycogen, which will meet the energy needs of that first period of what, to the body, is the start of a prolonged crisis. Adaptation must thereafter allow the mobilisation of the lipid and protein stores. Physiological priorities are the maintenance of blood glucose for brain function (for the starved person must be conscious enough to search for food and react to danger) and for rapid muscle movement (to chase more food and escape from equally hungry predators). This glucose can only be derived from gluconeogenesis using amino acids (and to a very small extent glycerol), and experiments have

Table 3   Reserves of Energy in a Normal Man

	Total in Body	Total Stores (in kg)	Energy Stores (kcal)
Carbohydrate	0·5	0·5	2 000
Protein	10	4	15 000
Fat	8	8	70 000

These are rounded off figures, for ease of handling. Women would in general have less supply all round and a greater proportion of fat. kcal are easier to work with; to obtain kJ, multiply by 4.2.

---

shown that about 60 g of protein per day is needed for this conversion. If it were used up at this rate over the whole period of starvation, the protein stores in our hypothetical man would last some 40 days.

Where does this protein come from, since there are no obvious anatomically sequestrated stores? In fact there is mobilisable protein in the gastrointestinal tract, the liver and the muscles. As the fast progresses, the pancreas regresses, and digestive enzymes are no longer synthesised. The liver cells are depleted of protein, the muscles atrophy, and the intestinal mucosa become paper thin. It is at this point that refeeding is dangerous, for if conducted too enthusiastically, it may cause inflammation and peritonitis.

Of course this 60 g protein, in energy terms, would yield only about 240 kcal per day. Even a small, starving man would need about 1800 kcal per day for survival, say another 1500 kcal on top of that provided by the protein. The balance comes from adipose tissue triglyceride, which supplies fatty acids to resting muscle, and ketone bodies to the brain. Although the brain is absolutely dependent on glucose, some of the requirement may be replaced by ketone bodies. In our hypothetical example the fat would last for

$$70\,000 \div 1500 = 45 \text{ days approximately}$$

or about the same as for the protein. Evidently, since both protein and fat are needed, the subject will die when one or the other runs out. Common observation indicates that fat varies more among individuals than protein. The fat stores are therefore a basic survival factor, the primaeval equivalent of the American Express Gold Card, and if an individual can build up enough adipose tissue to last out the protein supply, then he will survive for 40 days or so. An increment beyond the protein supply is of little use unless *in extremis* the brain can adapt to more and more ketosis, although we have little information on this situation in humans.

There are profound endocrine adaptations too. The secretion of insulin diminishes, and glucagon effects the mobilisation of fat, cortisol of protein. As substrates become scarce, there is yet another useful adaptation in the regression of the thyroid gland, further economising on substrates.

Perhaps most seriously, immunocompetence is compromised, and in the starving the actual cause of death is most often pneumonia or gastroenteritis.

The picture painted above is obviously modified a lot in the case of children, who tend on the whole to have lesser stores of all the substrates, even on a proportional basis, and perhaps to some extent in the case of women, who on average have a higher fat/protein ratio than men.

Of course medical names have been given to the phenomena surrounding starvation. **Marasmus** is merely another (Greek) word for starvation, and provides a convenient adjective in "marasmic". The other syndrome produces no convenient adjective but a descriptive noun, in **kwashiorkor**. A reading of the literature in the 1980s suggests that this entity, characterised by fatty liver, oedema and skin changes is not now so prominent. This may be because food is no longer contaminated with hepatotoxins (such as aflatoxins) but nobody knows its aetiology anyway.

SURGICAL PATIENTS

It it obvious enough why patients recovering from operations to the jaw and gastrointestinal tract become malnourished, but it came as a surprise when surveys done some years ago revealed a majority of unselected surgical patients to be decidedly marasmic. The reasons for this belong to a wider discussion of medical sociopathology but suffice it to remark here that biochemistry offers means by which the malnutrition can be detected. You can keep tabs on a number of proteins, like albumin, prealbumin and ferritin which will decrease rapidly in the serum as inanation progresses, but better is the creatinine-height index. Simply, in individuals the muscle mass as indexed by creatinine excretion should have a constant relationship to height, not weight, and in addition a reference interval (i.e. a standard for a population) for it can be worked out. Measuring it will detect marasmus in patients who do not appear to be particularly malnourished and who may maintain that they are eating well.

CACHEXIA OF CANCER

Again, it is easy to understand why patients with advanced cancer of the oesophagous, for example, should begin to look skeletal. But most cancer patients become thin, whatever the site. It appears they often lose their sense of smell and taste, and radiation and chemotherapy may also be culprits.

More fundamentally, is there any basis for saying that "Cancer feeds off the body" — a sort of long-standing folk message? The father of one of us swore that sixty years ago he saw a neighbour buy a fillet steak every day and press it on to some sort of maxillary cancer, and that when the steak was later removed its area of contact with the growth was white, drained of nourishment! It seems now that glutamine is released from the muscles of cancer patients, and since this is the form in which carbon is exported from muscles to fulfill energy requirements elsewhere, this idea may be some sort of analogy of the truth. At any rate, oncologists have learned that their patients do need nutritional support.

Breakdown of muscle protein is mediated at least in part by cachectin or tumour necrosis factor, the cytokine (Chap. 17a) first isolated from macrophages exposed to bacterial endotoxin.

ANOREXIA NERVOSA/BULIMIA NERVOSA

Everybody has now heard of anorexia nervosa. Novels deal with it (see Catherine Anne Howard's *Getting It Right*) and most people became aware when the singer Carol Carpenter died of it in the mid-eighties. It has even moved into the domain of telephone help agencies as one of the phone-in crises advertised by *Self Helpline* in London newspapers and magazines, along with sleeping problems and other more intimate matters. If severe, then the metabolic course is as outlined above, and the depletion of body fat usually has the further effect of amenorrhoea, leading some psychiatrists to speculate that the disease represents a flight from sexuality. It was Frisch who first pointed out, on the basis of studies of weight at menarche and dysmenorrhoea in female athletes, that a woman needs a certain amount of body fat (i.e. mobilisable energy) to support reproduction, and anorexics certainly fit that concept. There are however variants which present without obvious emaciation. A colleague tells me of the following case he saw.

"This girl, aged seventeen was brought into my surgery by her mother. 'She isn't right,' said the mother, 'she's always listless and lacks interest in everything and is not doing well at school. She never looks well'. I myself observed a very pale and thinnish but not actually emaciated young woman. I questioned her about what she was eating but the mother said she took the ordinary family fare, though not every day. Very little else could be elicited. I did a cursory physical examination, gave her some iron tablets, took some blood for the lab, and asked her to come back in a fortnight, indicating in as tactful a manner as possible that the mother's presence was not necessary on that occasion. The laboratory results were as follows. (The testing seems rather effusive, but it was partially funded by a body interested in adolescent medicine!)

| haemoglobin | 10.5 | g/100 ml | (reference interval,12–16) |
| iron | 5.1 | µmol/l | (6.6–26) |

ferritin	4.1	µg/l	(6–81)
glucose (random)	4.1	mmol/l	(4–7.8)
folate	11	nmol/l	(10–40)
vitamin B12	147	pmol/l	(150–700)
bicarbonate	37	mmol/l	(22–31)
potassium	2.9	mmol/l	(3.5–4.5)
sodium	134	mmol/l	(135–150)
creatinine	60	µmol/l	(62–106)
alanine transaminase	35	U/l	(0–40)
albumin	34	g/l	(39–50)
thyroxine (free)	25	pmol/l	(11.6–27)
thyroid stimulating hormone	1.3	mU/l	(0.4–4.5)

She had a hypochromic (iron deficiency) anaemia all right but that is so common as to be hardly worth remarking upon. The rather low albumin made one suspect some degree of malnutrition. Potassium was low and bicarbonate high. All else was essentially normal.

When she came back again I did a more thorough examination, again revealing nothing significant. I questioned her on her menstrual history but she was rather coy. On a hunch, I took a dental mirror and looked at the back of her teeth. Sure enough, the enamel was eroded. In the face of this, I induced her to admit to habitual self-induced vomiting after almost every meal. Gastric hydrochloric acid had been destructively pouring through the enamel. This also explained the low potassium and high bicarbonate — she was in state of chronic metabolic alkalosis and hypokalaemia due to the loss of the acid, potassium rich gastric juice. This is bulimia, or bulimia nervosa. It is sometimes characterised by purging rather than vomiting, and occasionally by both. After some ineffectual counselling on my part, she was referred to a psychiatrist and after a year or so is doing well."

INFORMATION FROM BOBBY SANDS

How long would a totally food-deprived castaway, refugee, anorexic or patient really survive? Despite the theoretical treatment above, indicating about 40 days for a 60 kg man, it is difficult to say. In this context there are no controlled experiments in humans. There is another group which do give relevant information, however, and these are the Irish republican prisoners who go on hunger strike. In 1916 Terence McSweeney, the Lord Mayor of Cork, starved himself to death over a period of 74 days. If this report is accurate, he must have had exceptional stores of protein and fat at the beginning of his ordeal. In more modern times, in 1981, four prisoners took the same course in Belfast and survived a mean of 62 days. Press photographs indicated that these were young men with no significant adiposity before the fast and so the inference is that metabolism slows down very considerably as it is prolonged, due to a relative hypothyroidism. Bobby Sands, the first to die, was said to be suffering from failing eyesight towards the end, presumably due to vitamin A deficiency. This was a surprise, since it has generally been supposed that the hypometabolism of starvation decreases the need for vitamins. These observations are valuable, but (it is to be hoped) the very last of their kind.

POSTSCRIPT

How does all this translate into patient care? The first lesson is that malnutrition may lurk unseen, especially in hospitalised patients, and even in some visitors to the office/surgery. But there are others — that those at risk of immunodeficiency must be provided with plenty of energy; that refeeding after starvation must be cautious. But perhaps the best example of applying this knowledge is the type of rough and ready calculation which may be required in the face of patient expectations. Suppose you **do** have an obese patient who swears, because he can no longer wheeze his way up the steps of a bus, that he will go on a total fast. (It is said, by the way, that fasting becomes not too painful after a while — the diminished secretion of gastric juices and digestive hormones at supposed mealtimes presumably ceases and thus quietens the gut. Or, shortage of neurotransmitters derived from nutrients damps down some brain activity. Also, is starvation not so painful for the old, as compared to the young? Popular tradition would certainly hold that young people suffer more.)

Suppose the hypothetical obese patient is 110 kg to start with. How long will it take him to reach a respectable 90 kg? The man will presumably not be very active, due to his obesity alone, and so you could assume an energy expenditure of about 2000 kcal per day. He will need to obtain almost all of this energy from fat after the first day of the fast he is determined to undertake, but will mobilise some protein for blood glucose, say 60 g per day giving 240 kcal; the remaining 1800 kcal is derived from fat, so in grams that is 1800/9 = 200 g fat per day, total substrate usage and so weight loss per day coming to 260 g, so far. But some further aspects have to be taken into account:

(1) There will be some obligatory loss of water with the protein, and to a lesser extent with the fat, so you could take a round of figure 400 g as the loss of weight, per day, to account for water too.

(2) Though theoretically the metabolic rate may slow down as he proceeds into the fast, due to relative hypothyroidism, if he really wants to lose weight he should try to maintain his job and lifestyle and for present purposes we can discount this factor.

(3) In a contrary sense, starving people seem to be able to utilise their substates more efficiently, that is, they are better able to conserve them as body mass and produce less wasteful heat on their oxidation. However this survival mechanism is difficult to quantitate.

So we are left with a working calculation, the desired weight loss divided by the calculated weight loss per day, or

$$20\,000 \div 400 = 50 \text{ days.}$$

That is the horrendous period over which he will have to go without food entirely to lose 20 kg! In fact, it is not certain that his protein stores will last that long, and he would be in great danger from hypoglycaemia and ketosis towards the end. He might more properly have a total fast of one month and then some protein and vitamin supplements, with a general check-up and review.

Further Reading

1. Garrow JS. Recent developments in clinical nutrition. *JRCP (Lond)* **23** : 15–21, 1989.
2. Frisch, R. Fatness, menarche, and female fertility. *Perspectives in Biol and Med* **28** : 611–633, 1985.

10b
Overweight and Overfat

"....... there were women in their late thirties and forties and older (women 'of a certain age'), all of them skin and bones (starved to near perfection). To compensate for the concupiscence missing from their juiceless ribs and atrophied backsides, they turned to the dress designers..."
— Tom Wolfe, **The Bonfire of the Vanities**

As the quotation implies, body shape, in so far as it can be manipulated by those with the means and the will to do so, is a function of social values, which tend to be mutable. Historically, the ideal (at least for women) has tended towards plumpness, as seen by inspection of the "venuses" of archaeological sites with their ponderous thighs and abdomens through the fleshy nudes of Rubens and Renoir in art galleries. Indeed in modern times, it has been established that a woman needs a certain amount of fat for reproductive activity, vide the loss of menses and other fertility problems in woman athletes and anorexics, so that the social value placed on adipose tissue probably had a biological rationale at base. Further, until about eighty years ago in Western Europe at least, leanness was associated with tuberculosis, plumpness freedom from it, but in the mid-twentieth century this ancient scourge largely disappeared, with the epidemic of heart disease and diabetes to a great extent replacing it. These modern epidemics are above all associated with obesity, and this no doubt contributed to a reversion of the old preference for fleshiness. But is the trend continuing? Fig. 30 charts the changing shape of female fashion models, who presumably represent an aspect of the current ideal, admittedly as modified by the ideas of dress designers. It seems that models are becoming ever more tubular, that is neither fatter nor leaner, but more like men!

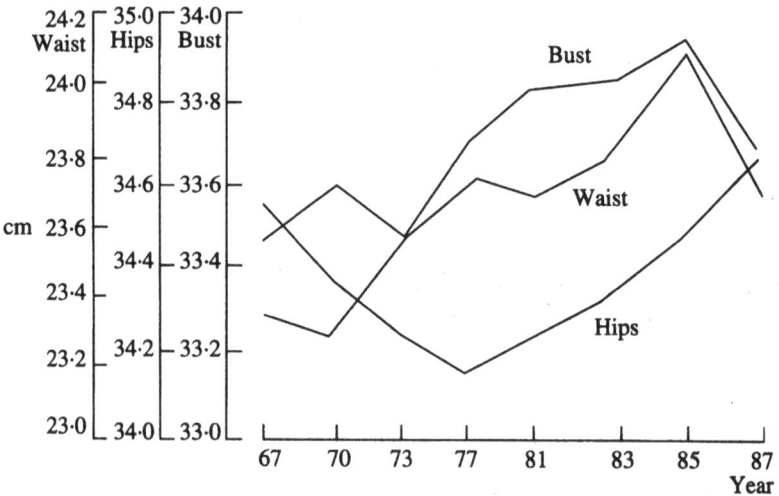

Fig. 30 The changing shapes of fashion models.

Drawn from the data in the paper by A Morris, T Cooper and PJ Cooper (*International Journal of Eating Disorders* **8** : 593–596, 1989.

A partial list of the conditions associated with obesity, in rough order of importance, is as follows:

(1) Diabetes
(2) Cerebrovascular disease
(3) Coronary heart disease
(4) Hypertension
(5) Accidents
(6) Respiratory disease
(7) Arthritis

The number of sufferers involved must be vast in any country.

WHAT IS OBESITY?

Obesity is important, but what is it? It is clear that it is not excess body weight per se. Body builders, for example, have large weights for their heights as compared to the rest of the populations they build within, yet they are quite obviously not obese. Obesity is an excess of adipose tissue over lean body mass, and is more accurately described as "overfat" than "overweight". However the term "putting on weight" rather than "putting on fat" is so ingrained we have to use it ourselves. All this still begs the question as to what is meant by "over". Are fat people just those who are a certain order of magnitude over the mean weight for height, or do they represent a sub-population identifiable by a specific pathology? Opinion has tended to favour the former, following efforts by life insurance companies, particularly the Metropolitan Life Insurance Company of New York; by actuarial calculation, it established the risk of death associated with various strata of body weight. Of course if you want an insurance policy you must submit to a medical examination, so your weight and height are recorded at that time, then the insurance company records your survival time thereafter. The calculations of survival (which did not initially distinguish between overweight and overfat) were criticised on the grounds that the section of the population seeking life insurance is atypical — it is more prudent, or more anxious, certainly more wealthy than the norm. And without doubt, women were underrepresented, not being breadwinners and needing policies at the time the pioneering studies were conducted.

Later work however has tended in general to bear out the validity of the actuarial calculations, with no significant differences being found between men and women. If the general trend towards greater mortality with increasing weight is established, quantitating it remains controversial. The relevant figures are found at the backs of medical and nutritional books, in the form of "ideal weights" (now more usually called "desirable weights") for height, and which must be attained to minimise the risk of premature morbidity/mortality. They used to be engraved in aluminium plaques on penny weighing machines, when such were still found on railway station platforms — the modern electronic weighing devices do not have room for them. The tables are usually divided into sectors for small, medium and large frames, the definition of which you have to decide for yourself. Ancel Keys (Ref. 1 below) has written that these are all armchair concoctions starting with questionable assumptions. Recently an attempt has been made to put frame size on a scientific basis by measuring the width of the elbow bones. An equally sophisticated but at the same time simpler approach is to measure the Quetelet or body mass index, namely weight over height squared (kg/m). This corrects the body weight with the square of the height — using the squared denominator tends to eliminate the lean tissue inevitably associated with increasing height and allow comparison of adiposity itself, and there is no separation of men and women using such an index. The Royal College of Physicians suggests that obesity starts when the Quetelet index rises to over 30. That is, if I am a fairly normal height for a man, say 5 feet 11 inches, (1.8 m) I should not let my weight rise above 80 kg giving an index of

$$80 \div 1.8 = 26$$

(26 being a more acceptable figure than the 30 definitely establishing obesity.)

For all that, there is evidence that in old age a degree of overweight, however defined, is a protective factor.

BIOCHEMICAL REASONING AND OBESITY

The reasons why some people carry around large amounts of adipose tissue, while others are in comparison very lean have not been clarified at this date. It has been established, however, in spite of popular belief, that fat people as a whole eat no more than their lean companions, and usually much less. There is evidently a set-point for adults in health, lasting for years and sometimes decades, governed by the balance between energy intake and utilisation, and which is only disturbed under extreme circumstances, such as disease, starvation and gorging. The set point may be maintained by:

(1) Genetic factors: twin studies, particularly of the very efficient Danish Twin Register, show that there is a distinct genetic component.

(2) Modulation of uncoupled electron transport. If electron transport generates merely heat instead of ATP, the basis for the synthesis of all tissue components, then the energy in foodstuffs is merely dissipated. This type of uncoupled respiration is thought to be characteristic of the mitochondria of brown fat, which may persist into adult life in some subjects. (There is plenty of it in babies to allow non-shivering thermogenesis.) In a word, if substrates, even in excess, can be switched to brown fat deposits in a controlled manner then weight can be kept constant.

(3) Fat cell signalling. One theory supposes that fat cells, which on mobilisation of their lipid droplets can shrink to one thousandth of their original volume, are able to signal to the brain that they are in such a dangerous condition, and make feeding an urgent biological imperative. The signalling device, if it exists, is however unknown. It also seems that fat cells can be created but not destroyed; so if there is gorging or gross overfeeding at some stage the new cells, even if subsequently depleted of their lipid, are always there ready to be refilled. This is known as the *ratchet effect*.

(4) Modulation of lipoprotein lipase, the enzyme first encountered in Chap. 4a as releasing fatty acids from chylomicrons and VLDL, to allow these fatty acids to be assimilated into muscle and adipose tissue. Evidently, if this enzyme is overactive in some way there will be gain of adipose tissue. It must therefore be exquisitely modulated to replete adipose tissue but not overfill it in the interests of operating the set-point efficiently. One modulator is insulin, but there must be others. Ovariectomy, for example, decreases lipoprotein lipase activity.

A curious feature of lipoprotein lipase is its different activity from one locale to another — it is thought to be more active round the hips and legs in women — that is, in the places they tend to lay down fat; in contrast maximum activity in men is in the abdominal region. One thing is certain, the doctor or scientist who learns to manipulate lipoprotein lipase activity in specific regions but not others will become famous and make a fortune!

What lessons can be carried over from the basic sciences, and biochemistry in particular, in the interests of treating the obese? The first and most important is that nobody can obviate the first law of thermodynamics. If you eat food of an energy content in excess of your expenditure, you may or may not put on fat, depending on the circumstances and the robustness of the set-point, but if you eat food of less energy than you need for daily existence, you **must** lose weight. The second biochemical point is that all the major substrates in foods can yield adipose tissue triglycerides. The efficiency with which this can be accomplished is however different. One gram of ingested triglyceride can be converted almost quantitatively to depot fat — it needs only to be rearranged with respect to its fatty acid composition. One gram of carbohydrate has to be converted to fat by a tortuous process, involving energy-demanding phosphorylation and production of two and three carbon units for fatty acids and glycerol respectively (Fig. 31). Probably at best only about 0.3 g fat can be synthesised from the starting 1 g of carbohydrate. Protein probably yields even less. It follows that for losing weight (in the presence of a sufficiently intense energy expenditure as physical work/sport) a high carbohydrate/ low fat diet is preferable. Why not a high protein diet? Apart form its intrinsic expense, there is evidence that human beings cannot for long tolerate a diet of almost entirely lean meat, or fish. Suggesting this sort of diet to a patient may

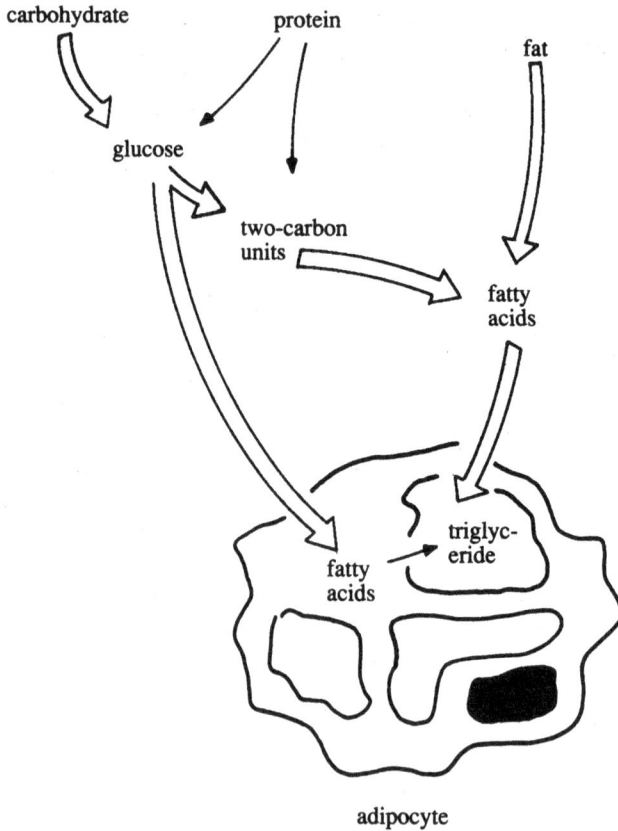

Fig. 31   The flow of substrates into adipose tissue.

The contribution from protein would be minor in most if not all circumstances. Since there is no glycerol kinase in the adipocyte the glycerol needed for triglyceride synthesis is also derived from incoming glucose, rather than from glycerol released by lipoprotein lipase at the endothelial surface of the adipose tissue capillaries.

produce a favourable reaction but in the long run will be a waste of time. Indeed there is some evidence that most human beings have an innate craving for carbohydrates when deprived of them, sometimes known as "carboholism."

The problem, as Prof McGilvery put it, is that man is an omnivore, and the composition of the diet can fluctuate wildly. Thus (as he writes) "man ... may be gulping down the still-warm hindquarters of a wild pig (1.5% carbohydrate, 25% fat, 16% protein) brought down by a spear to provide the week's ration, while aspiring to a life of self-contemplation in a land of milk (4.9% carbohydrate, 3.9% fat, and 3.5 % protein) and honey (79 % carbohydrate, 3% fat, 0% protein)."

Like Oscar Wilde, most people can resist everything but temptation. Doctors who consistently try to treat obesity are said to count among the most frustrated individuals you will encounter anywhere.

Further Reading

1. Keys, A. Overweight, obesity, coronary heart disease, and mortality. *Nutr Rev* **38** : 297–307, 1980.
2. Truswell AS. Obesity: diagnosis and risks. *Br Med J* **291** : 655–658, 1985.
3. Bjorntorp P. How should obesity be defined? *J Intern Med* **227** : 147–149, 1990.

PART THREE

Control Mechanisms and Clinical Practice

11a

Fluoride: The Diagnostician's Friend

Outwith haematology, the measurement of glucose is still the most frequently requested laboratory procedure — whether or not the patient is diabetic it is a component of most screens and profiles. Other conditions for which it is part of the request panel are as follows (some of them being coextensive):

(1) Inherited disorders (e.g glycogen storage and others).
(2) Pituitary disorders (acromegaly, Cushing's syndrome).
(3) Adrenal cortex disorders (Cushing's disease).
(4) Hypoglycaemic states (insulinoma, reactive hypoglycaemia).
(5) Kidney disorders (proximal tubular defects).
(7) Liver diseases (cirrhosis, Reye's syndrome).

Whatever the suspected condition, the measurement of glucose must be accurate — for example, the diagnosis of diabetes, in the absence of florid signs and symptoms, is made on rather narrow criteria (see Chap. 1a), and in connection with most of the other items in the list above, decisions may also have to be taken on the basis of small changes.

The trouble is that in shed blood, glucose starts to disappear very rapidly, due to the vigorous glycolysis of the red blood cells. However, ways to circumvent this are available:

(1) The blood may be immediately deproteinised, which removes the glycolytic enzymes.
(2) The blood may be taken into a heparinised syringe, and the cells may be removed from the plasma immediately, that is without waiting for the blood to clot.
(3) The blood may be drawn into a syringe charged with an inhibitor of glycolysis.

(1) and (2) above are difficult to achieve in routine practice. When you are taking blood from a series of patients, it is logistically almost impossible to process each specimen immediately. Most authorities favour number 3.

USE OF ENOLASE INHIBITORS FOR ACCURATE BLOOD GLUCOSE

If we can remind ourselves (yet again) of the key steps in glycolysis (Fig. 32), it is obvious that it comprises a large number of enzymic steps, and any of these could be inhibited to prevent the disappearance of glucose, on the general principle that breaking down a production line at any point blocks the whole process. The most convenient point of interruption however happens to be at the enolase reaction, for this enzyme has been known for many decades to be inhibited by fluoride.

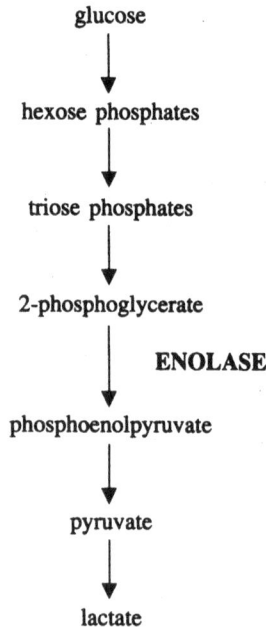

glucose

↓

hexose phosphates

↓

triose phosphates

↓

2-phosphoglycerate

↓ **ENOLASE**

phosphoenolpyruvate

↓

pyruvate

↓

lactate

Fig. 32   A reminder of the key steps in glycolysis.

It is the enolase step which is inhibited by fluoride ions.

VIGNETTE

You are supervising the casualty department of a hospital on a busy evening. At about 9.30 the ambulancemen bring in a comatose patient, an elderly lady found in the street. There is no smell of alcohol on the breath, and no outward sign of injury.

The patient seems somewhat dehydrated — sunken eyes and parchmentlike skin — and diabetic coma seems more than likely. A urine specimen for glycosuria is indicated but of course under the circumstances is difficult to obtain. You ask the nurse to take blood for a diabetic panel and to mark the form STAT, before moving on to an incoming heart attack. The results come back in about one and a half hours and are as follows:

glucose	10.6	mmol/l	(reference interval 4–7.8)
sodium	133	mmol/l	(135–150)
potassium	3.5	mmol/l	(3.5–5)
creatinine	512	μmol/l	(62–106)
bicarbonate	18	mmol/l	(22–31)
urea	11	mmol/l	(2.5–6.4)
chloride	94	mmol/l	(101–111)

There is evidence of an increased anion gap here, i.e.

$$(Na^+ + K^+) - (Cl^- + bicarbonate^-)$$

is about 25, whereas the normal should be about 16. Thus there is the suggestion of ketosis consistent with a diabetic crisis, but the glucose is probably to be considered normal, for you do not know if the patient is postprandial or not. There is a condition called normoglycaemic ketoacidosis, but it is rather rare and it would be unwise to plump for it at this stage. Another reason for the anion gap might be lactic acidosis but a request for a STAT lactic acid still leaves you with a wait of about an hour, so having put into train the tests for the heart case you ask the nurse what syringe was used to take the blood from the elderly lady. Unfortunately, with the nurse harassed and new to the job, it turns out to have been a plain one, not the fluoridated one. Hurriedly, another specimen is taken in a fluoridated syringe (the third in an hour, but anyway the patient is unconscious) and taken directly up to the lab by hand. The result, phoned down, is 18.4 mmol/l. You are then fairly confident of the diagnosis of diabetic ketoacidosis, and infusion of low dose insulin/potassium brings the patient out of danger. In fact the glucose is still not high enough to lead you to expect a coma, but the creatinine and urea results suggest long-term kidney damage, so the patient is probably not handling the acid load from the ketones as well as might be expected in a younger and possibly better controlled subject.

OTHER USES OF FLUORIDE

One of the theories of the efficacy of fluoride in preventing dental caries is that it inhibits glycolysis in acid-producing bacteria. However, here we focus on other analyses which may need preliminary inhibition of glycolysis in the erythrocyte. First of all, there is lactic acid, which can disappear due to conversion to pyruvate in oxidising conditions, as when there is a head of air in the syringe. Moreover, red blood cells with their vigorous glycolysis can produce quite large amounts of lactic acid unless they are separated from the serum or plasma at a very early stage after the blood is drawn. So in the vignette above, if the lactate specimen had also been taken in a plain tube, the result might equally have been misleading.

Pyruvate estimations may need a fluoridated tube for the converse reason, that is it can be converted to lactate in shed blood, but since it is thought to be an even more labile substance than glucose or lactate then the laboratory is generally called upon to provide a perchlorate deproteinising solution to receive the blood the moment it is drawn. That is manoeuvre number 1 above.

Alcohol is the other substance measured in blood drawn into a fluoridated tube. The reasons for this are not so simple. A glance at Fig. 47 reveals that alcohol is not removed by glycolysis. It may be that if glycolysis is inhibited by fluoride at the enolase stage, which is rather late in the sequence, then any NAD present will be converted to NADH in the glyceraldehyde phosphate dehydrogenase reaction. NAD is necessary for the conversion of alcohol to form acetaldehyde (Chap. 18c), so its removal will preserve the alcohol.

But however you rationalise the use of fluoride in this situation, if you are a police surgeon and take the specimen in the wrong syringe, then the analytical results will be inadmissible in court.

Comment

The above might seem to be a string of technicalities. Be that as it may, you have to understand such technicalities to avoid disasters.

Further Reading

1. Chan AYW, Swaminatham R and Cockram CS. Effectiveness of sodium fluoride as a preservative of glucose in blood. *Clin Chem* **35** : 315–317, 1989.
2. Burrin JM and Alberti KGMM. What is blood glucose: can it be measured? *Diabetic Medicine* **7** : 199–206, 1990.

11b

HMG-CoA Reductase Inhibitors

In Chapter 4a we discussed the thorny question of high serum cholesterol concentrations, mainly with reference to aberrant low density lipoprotein (LDL) receptors in the condition familial hypercholesterolaemia (FH). Not all cases of primary hypercholesterolaemia are due to this disorder however — an alternative diagnosis is polygenic or common hypercholesterolaemia, which may be defined as raised LDL cholesterol unattributable to a known single genetic defect. In it, serum cholesterol may not be so elevated as in FH and usually tendon xanthomata do not occur. Nevertheless, polygenic hypercholesterolaemia carries about a 2–3 times enhanced risk of coronary heart disease.

Mammalian cells have the capacity to synthesise cholesterol from acetate molecules (Fig. 33); cholesterol is an essential substance for the maintenance of membrane structure and as a precursor both of steroid hormones and bile acids. The rate limiting enzyme in cholesterol synthesis is β-hydroxy-β-methylglutaryl CoA reductase (HMG-CoA reductase), which catalyses the conversion of β-hydroxy-β-methylglutaryl-CoA to mevalonic acid. When a cell is actively making cholesterol there is an increase in HMG-CoA reductase expression but conversely, when sufficient cholesterol is available, there is a mechanism available to prevent its uneccessary accumulation. Firstly, there is a reduction in HMG-CoA reductase activity, thus reducing *de novo* synthesis. Secondly, free cholesterol is esterified to form cholesterol ester through the action of intracellular acyl-CoA cholesterol acyltransferase (ACAT). Another regulating process, which was discussed in Chap. 4a, is the reduction in the expression of LDL receptors at the cell surface thus limiting uptake of cholesterol-rich LDL particles.

A number of clinical trials have shown that pharmacologically reducing raised plasma cholesterol will reduce the risk of coronary heart disease risk. Broadly speaking for every 1% decrease in plasma cholesterol achieved, a corresponding 2% reduction in coronary risk is observed. One of the earliest and biggest was the World Health Organisation trial of about 16 000 subjects with raised serum cholesterol, in which clofibrate was used to successfully lower cholesterol over a five-year period. Unfortunately although this drug — which lowers cholesterol by increasing the activity of lipoprotein lipase and also increasing LDL clearance — reduced myocardial infarction deaths, there was an increase in non-cardiovascular

two-carbon units

↓

acetoacetyl CoA

↓

β-hydroxy-β-methylglutaryl CoA
(HMG CoA)

|

HMG CoA REDUCTASE

↓

mevalonic acid

↓

isoprenoids

↓

squalene

↓

lanosterol

↓

cholesterol

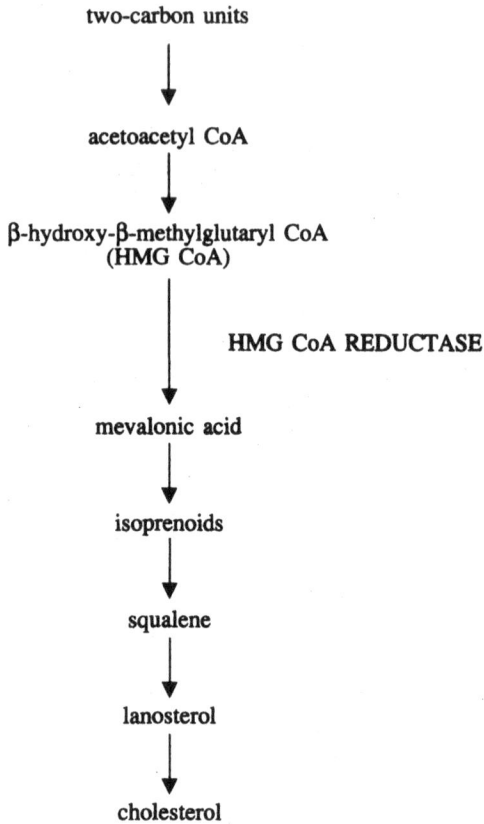

Fig. 33 A summary of cholesterol synthesis.

The reductase step is rate limiting.

morbidity and mortality. Notably too, there were significantly more cholecystectomies performed in treated subjects as compared to placebo subjects.

The double blind Coronary Drug Project (CDP) trial looked at a number of drug therapies in the treatment of 3908 hypercholesterolaemic males but specifically found niacin (a nicotinic acid derivative that can lower cholesterol by reducing LDL synthesis and probably also by enhancing lipoprotein lipase) to reduce total mortality by about 11% more than the placebo-treated group, this being associated with a 10% reduction of serum cholesterol.

In the Lipid Research Clinics Coronary Primary Prevention Trial, cholestyramine was used in a study of 3806 males with hypercholesterolaemia, over approximately seven and a half years. The major end-points of this trial were nonfatal myocardial infarction and death from coronary heart disease, which were reduced by 19% in the cholestyramine-treated group along with a reduction in serum cholesterol of about 9%. Strangely however, overall mortality was similar in both the placebo and cholestyramine-treated groups. Cholestyramine is an anion-exchange resin which binds bile salts in the large intestine and causes their elimination in the faeces. This causes clearance of the steroid nucleus from the body and so increases the uptake of cholesterol by the liver for the synthesis of more bile salts, with a concomitant fall in serum cholesterol. There is an observable enhancement of LDL receptor expression at the hepatocyte plasma membrane to facilitate LDL cholesterol uptake from the serum.

Yet another study was the Helsinki Heart Study, in which 4081 middle-aged males with hypercholesterolaemia were treated with gemfibrozil (a phenoxyisobutyrate derivative similar in action to clofibrate) for a five-year period. There was a 34% reduction in coronary episodes events in the drug-treated group and a 8% reduction in serum cholesterol despite a similar total mortality in the two study groups.

"STATINS"

Although dietary control and use of the drugs mentioned above can be used to treat hypercholesterolaemia, the multiplicity of undesirable side effects of the latter has made further therapeutic strategies highly desirable, and a recent development has been the use of HMG-CoA reductase inhibitors. By inhibiting cholesterogenesis in the liver, they reduce intracellular cholesterol and promote LDL receptor expression in an adaptation to allow more LDL uptake, clearance of LDL from the circulation and lowering of plasma cholesterol. There is also evidence that the HMG-CoA reductase inhibitors can slightly increase the so-called cardioprotective lipoprotein particles, the high-density lipoproteins (HDL), although no significant effect is observed for serum triglyceride.

The family of drugs developed that inhibit HMG-CoA reductase have been given the suffix "statin". One such is lovastatin which was first available on prescription in the United States, the equivalent in Europe being simvastatin. These drugs are marketed for the treatment of raised cholesterol in primary hypercholesterolaemia. The scale of this problem, if it is a problem, is demonstrated by the estimated sales of $2000 million of just one proprietary brand by 1992.

Full evaluation of the "statins" is awaited, and some concern has been expressed over side-effects such as a myositis-like syndrome characterised by raised blood creatine kinase levels, or even rhabdomyolysis, that is severe muscle breakdown leading to the liberation of myocyte products which can damage the renal tubules and lead to renal failure. There are also abnormalities in liver function tests, by way of raised serum transaminase activity in some patients. The long-term effects of inhibiting cholesterol synthesis in humans are also largely unknown, and need investigation, particularly as mevalonic acid is the precursor not only of the steroid hormones and bile salts but also ubiquinone (the mediator of electron transport) and dolichol (a precursor of glycoprotein saccharides).

ILLUSTRATIVE CASE HISTORY

A 52-year-old bank manager went to his family doctor because he was concerned about swellings on his elbows and the fact that his wife thought he had "strange rings" in his eyes. A family history revealed that his father and brother had both died in their fifties from "heart attacks". Physical examination was unremarkable except for confirming the nodular protruberances, that is xanthomas, on both elbows and the bilateral arcus senilis. The general practitioner asked the patient to come to see him the next morning before having breakfast and took a blood sample for dispatch to the laboratory. Two or three days later he obtained the following results.

cholesterol	10.9	mmol/l	(reference interval, < 5.2)
triglyceride	1.7	mmol/l	(0.5–1.8)
HDL-cholesterol	0.9	mmol/l	(0.75–1.73)

The only feature of interest is the high blood cholesterol, which is almost entirely due to LDL cholesterol. We can infer this because HDL cholesterol is low, and triglycerides are normal, meaning that there can be little contribution to the total cholesterol from VLDL. If required, there can be formal calculation of LDL cholesterol by the Friedwald formula:

$$\text{LDL cholesterol} = \text{total cholesterol} - \frac{\text{triglycerides}}{2.2} - \text{HDL cholesterol}$$

The first thing to do here is to check for any secondary cause of the hypercholesterolaemia, which does however seem unlikely in view of the family history as related. However other causes could be:

(1) Biliary obstruction
(2) Nephrotic syndrome
(3) Hypothyroidism

Some careful further testing was necessary to eliminate these, leaving a genetically determined hypercholesterolaemia as the only possible diagnosis. The patient was introduced to a low cholesterol, low saturated fat, high fibre diet and over a period of months achieved a lowering of the serum cholesterol to about 8.4 mmol/l, but this was considered to be still too high and he was started on a bile-acid binding agent. Unfortunately this caused embarrassing flatulence and he refused to continue. Consequently a HMG-CoA reductase inhibitor was tried after base-line liver and renal function tests, as well as the muscle enzyme creatine kinase, were performed. These were all normal. The inhibitor had reduced the serum cholesterol further, to 5.9 mmol/l, at the latest lipid clinic appointment, and this was considered to be highly satisfactory.

Further Reading

1. Illingworth DR. HMG CoA reductase inhibitors. *Curr Opin Lipidology* **2** : 24–30, 1991.
2. Davey-Smith G. and Pekkanen J. Should there be a moratorium on the use of cholesterol lowering drugs? *Br Med J* **304** : 431–433, 1992.
3. Grundy SM. HMG CoA reductase inhibitors for treatment of hypercholesterolaemia. *N Eng J Med* **319** : 24–33, 1988.

11c
ACES Go Places

That the kidney may be important in hypertension was evident from the oft-cited experiments of Goldblatt, who in the thirties observed a raised blood pressure when he removed one kidney of a dog and constricted the renal artery of the other. Almost fifty years previously it had been shown that kidney extract contains a particularly powerful vasoconstricting compound which, over the passage of time, was ascribed the name angiotensin. The biochemical pathways involving this compound have become well researched recently, especially with the advent of a new class of drug, namely the angiotensin converting enzyme inhibitors, ACE inhibitors for short, which have a salient part to play in the management of patients with hypertension and cardiac failure.

CLEAVAGES

The role of angiotensinogen demonstrates the manner in which a relatively inactive large molecule can be cleaved to form small highly potent molecules.

Angiotensinogen is a glycoprotein of about 400 amino acid residues, synthesised mainly in the liver under the stimulus of glucocorticoids and oestrogens. By means of the proteolytic activity of renin, another glycoprotein found in substantial amounts in the juxtaglomerular apparatus of the kidney, angiotensinogen can be cleaved to form a decapeptide called angiotensin I. This prohormone then undergoes conversion to the active hormone, angiotensin II, via further proteolytic cleavage in the lungs, by angiotensin converting enzyme (ACE), in a process which removes the dipeptide histidine-leucine from the carboxyl group end of angiotensin I. Angiotensin II, which is therefore an octapeptide, can in turn be converted to a relatively inactive compound angiotensin III by removal of the N-terminal aspartate residue, catalysed by the enzyme aminopeptidase. Further smaller degradation compounds may also be formed through the action of angiotensinases, as in Fig. 34.

As has already been mentioned that the protease renin is released from the juxtaglomerular cells associated with the afferent renal arteriole and in close prox-

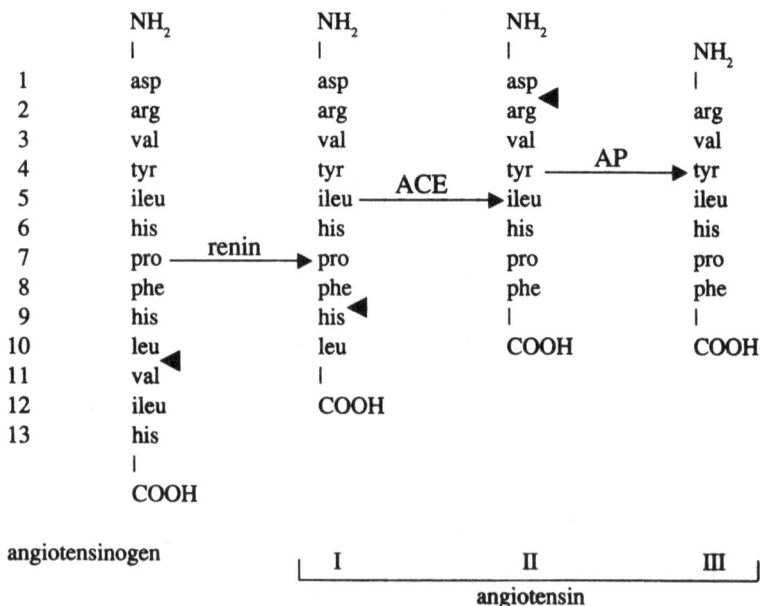

Fig. 34   The activation of angiotensinogen.

Angiotensin I has limited biological activity but the subsequent cleavages angiotensin converting enzyme (ACE) and aminopeptidase (AP) give powerfully hypertensive peptides.

imity to the macula densa cells. Control of renin secretion is important in that normally it is the rate limiting enzyme of the renin-angiotensin system, and incorporates a variety of different physiological mechanisms, as follows:

(1) Chemical control of sodium ion concentration sensed by chemoreceptors of the macula densa. Renin is released in hyponatraemia as a signal of hypovolaemia.

(2) Renal afferent arteriole vascular stretch sensed by baroreceptors in the proximity of the juxtaglomerular cells. Thus hypovolaemia may again be expected to evoke renin release.

(3) Sympathetic nervous system activity sensed by neural control systems involving beta receptors, also in the close vicinity of the juxtaglomerular cells.

It is thus evident that there is multifactorial control of the renin-angiotensin system, emphasing its importance in pressor homeostasis. The actions of angiotensin II are accordingly diverse. It is:

(1) A very potent vasoconstricting hormone.

(2) An effector for the release of aldosterone from the adrenal glands.

(3) An enhancer of sympathetic nervous system activation.

INTERACTIONS

Also of interest is the interaction of the renin-angiotensin system with the bradykinin system and, in addition, the atrial natriuretic peptides. Bradykinin is an inflammatory mediator, produced from its own precursor bradykininogen, which is cleaved by the enzyme kallikrein. Not only can bradykinin evoke vasodilatation, it can also enhance prostaglandin formation. ACE is known to inactivate bradykinin and thus ACE inhibitors would be expected to potentiate it. Atrial natriuretic peptide, released from cardiac atrial tissue in part by the effect of atrial stretch receptors which reflect blood volume status, can inhibit aldosterone secretion and thus sodium retention and also the release of renin. It is therefore antagonistic to the renin-angiotensin system.

From this it may be evident that inhibitors of the renin-angiotensin pathway may have some therapeutic use in conditions in which the renin-angiotensin system is over-expressed. Illnesses in which this would be of possible benefit include some cases of hypertension, where increased vasoconstriction and sodium retention can occur, and congestive cardiac failure where a vasodilating effect and reduction of fluid retention would be of importance in reducing the work of the heart.

The pharmacological quest for ACE inhibitors has been an extensive one, resulting in a number of suitable agents, the most established being captopril, enalapril and lisinopril. ACE is a zinc containing peptidase structurally similar to carboxypeptidase, but more specific as regarding substrate recognition, requiring only a free carboxylic acid residue at the carboxyl end of the polypeptide, provided proline is absent from the penultimate position.

The zinc ion at the active site of ACE is important for the binding to peptide substrates and has been the target for drug "attack". Captopril posseses a sulphydryl group capable of binding tightly to the ion, thus inhibiting the enzyme. Conversely however enalapril and lisinopril utilise a "strategically" placed carboxyl group to interact with the zinc. Biochemical elucidation of the active site ACE has thus enabled molecular maneouvering to target drug-induced inhibition.

The structural differences between these ACE inhibitors can also explain some of their side-effects. The sulphydryl group of captopril has been implicated, for example, in the bizarre taste of metal in the mouth (ageusia) experienced by some patients. In addition this sulphydryl group has been postulated as being important in the association of nephrotic syndrome and membranous glomerulonephritis seen in some patients on high dose captopril, which has been less frequently reported in users of other ACE inhibitors lacking the sulphydryl group. Captopril does have a possible advantage over the abovementioned ACE inhibitors in that it has a shorter half-life, which may have some therapeutic relevance.

Other side-effects elicited by ACE inhibitors as a whole can be worked out from the physiological actions of angiotensin. Hypotension can be precipitous, and hyponatraemia and hyperkalaemia can occur. Some side-effects can be ascribed to the impaired breakdown of bradykinin, which may precipitate angioedema in susceptible individuals. Angioedema is an acute non-pitting oedema of mucous membranes and skin in which involvement of the larynx or tongue can result in fatal obstruction of the respiratory tract. Presumably bradykinin is involved because of its vasodilating and increased tissue permeability actions. Interestingly, sensitivity to bradykinin may be important as the cause of the dry, irritating cough that possibly as many as one in eight patients on ACE inhibitors experience.

But a too gloomy picture of ACE inhibitors is not appropriate as they are clearly providing useful ammunition for clinicians in the treatment of hypertension and cardiac failure. Results of the Cooperative North Scandinavian Enalapril Survival Study (Consensus Study) have been so encouraging that one editorial stated that, in the case of certain chronic heart failure, patients: "To prescribe a diuretic and to delay ACE inhibitor therapy is no longer supportable".

Further Reading

1. Roberts CJC. Role of angiotensin converting enzyme inhibitors in the management of hypertension and heart failure. *Rec Adv Cardiol* **10** : 175–200, 1987.
2. Braunwald E. ACE inhibitors , a cornerstone of the treatment of heart failure. *The N Engl J Med* **325** : 351–353, 1991.

12a

Calcium: The Medium and the Messenger

Look at the back of any medical textbook for the list of biochemical "reference intervals" (or "normal values" if the writers are on the conservative side). Glucose in serum can range over a concentration of 4 mmol/l (4 to 8, say) and still be considered non-pathological; enzymes can vary widely in the normal subject, for example 0–40 U/l is representative for aspartate transaminase, or AST. But look at the calcium entry. The range for healthy people is generally put at about 2.2–2.6 mmol/l. However, it is established that about half the calcium in serum is physiologically inactive, as it is bound to proteins and to inorganic anions like citrate, and the range for the ionised or active calcium is narrower still, 1.13–1.32 mmol/l. This implies that it is very tightly homeostatically controlled, and we may infer that its concentration is critical, not so much because of its role in bone formation, but for its importance as a messenger in cell function. Indeed, it has a central role in the contraction of all forms of muscle, the secretion of exocrine, endocrine and neurocrine products, and the breakdown of glycogen.

THE CALCIUM PARTITION SYSTEM

In the cell cytosol, ionised calcium exists in the range 100–200 nmol/l, whereas in the extracellular fluid, it is 500–10 000 times that concentration. It is clear that homeostasis inside the cell is if anything tighter than in the serum. The gradient is maintained by two mechanisms, the $Ca^{2+}/2H^+$ ATPase, or calcium pump, and the $3Na^+/Ca^{2+}$ exchanger. In the stimulated state, in glucagon mediated glycogen breakdown for example, there is an influx of calcium across the plasma membrane, and the intracellular concentration rises. The calcium binding protein calmodulin then modulates the relevant changes in metabolic activity of the stimulated cell; however, since the effects of the stimulation must be reversed to allow a new state of receptivity, the calmodulin itself reactivates the calcium pump in the interests of the original gradient.

Muscle is a little different in that there is an intracellular calcium partitioning system, the sarcoplasmic reticulum releasing stored calcium into the cytoplasm when muscle is electrically stimulated. However, calmodulin again detects the rise and restores the resting state via the calcium pump.

In mitochondria, calcium uptake is also an energy linked function and indeed comparatively massive amounts can be accumulated; this appears to protect the cell as a whole from calcium overaccumulation.

The mechanisms controlling influx and efflux are robust but can of course be overwhelmed. Rapid release of calcium from bone, for example, or calcium intoxication due to pica (eating chalk or cheese; they are not all that different, in fact, they both loaded with calcium) will compromise the partitioning of the ion between the extracellular and intracellular fluids. Hypercalcaemia (or for that matter hypocalcaemia) is always a circumstance to be investigated thoroughly. And as mentioned above, it needs only small shifts, less than 1 mmol/l, for calcium to become pathologically high or low.

Unexplained Hypercalcaemia

Some of the causes of hypercalcaemia may be listed as:
(1) Skeletal metastases
(2) PTH hypersecretion, ectopic or eutopic
(3) PTH-like factors in malignancy
(4) Renal failure
(5) Sarcoidosis and other granulomatous disorders
(6) Myeloma
(7) Malignant hyperthermia
(8) Neonatal hypercalcaemia
(9) Vitamin D toxicity
(10) Acromegaly
(11) Thiazide diuretics

Initially suspicion will rest upon the most common causes, hyperparathyroidism and malignancy. These are dealt with in Chap. 14b in relation to endocrine problems; here we wish to deal with some other aspects. The list above also includes kidney problems and enhanced absorption (vitamin D toxicity). Sarcoidosis, a disease still of puzzling aetiology, involving granulomatous lesions in diverse parts of the body, is associated with an unexplained vitamin D sensitivity.

The hypercalcaemic patient may be symptomless, but may also feel generaly ill; there may be lethargy, personality changes, anorexia, polyuria, cardiac arrhythmia, hypertension, kidney stomes, and joint pains. In one form of hypercalcaemia there is an often fatal rise in body temperature, as below.

MALIGNANT HYPERTHERMIA

Malignant hyperthermia or malignant hyperpyrexia is an inherited, pharmacological ("pharmacogenetic") condition linked to calcium metabolism. After induction of anaesthesia, the susceptible subject begins to exhibit a very rapid rise in temperature. There is a striking acidosis and carbon dioxide accumulation in the blood, with calcium, magnesium, and phosphate, also being raised. Among the enzymes, the most striking increase is seen in creatine kinase activity, with the skeletal muscle-associated MM isoenzyme being the most prominent. There is also a heavy myoglobinuria. The rapid rise in temperature can only be accounted for by some metabolic activity in muscle — it consists of about 40% of the body mass, and no other tissue could generate so much heat. The rise in serum CK-MM and urine myoglobin confirms muscle involvement. It was shown some years ago by direct experiment that during the hyperthermic crisis there is a release of calcium into the myoplasm from sarcoplasmic reticulum. This results in:

(1) Prolonged contraction and rigidity
(2) Activation of glycogen phosphorylase
(3) Catastrophic rise in temperature

Thus the heat production caused by oversupply of calcium is at the same time fuelled by glycogen breakdown for the same reason (Fig. 35).

In one case reported, a young man was in hospital for minor orthopaedic surgery. Under general anaesthesia with halothane, he was noted to have cardiac arrhythmia which however responded to lignocaine (a local anaesthetic also useful in ventricular arrhythmias). Shortly after that, however, the heart rate increased dramatically and the anaesthetist became aware — merely by touching — of a rise in the patient's skin temperature. The nasopharyngeal temperature, which is more informative than that of the axilla, was then monitored and found to be no less than 43 degrees; at the same time the blood gas results showed a marked acidosis. The creatine kinase (total) at this time was about 4000 U/l (reference interval 60–370 U/l). The ionised calcium was 1.56 mmol/l (reference interval, 1.13–1.32).

The anaesthetist was by now well aware that he was dealing with malignant hyperthermia, ice-packs were applied, and cold saline was even infused into the stomach. Dantrolene (a diffuse muscle relaxant) proved ineffective and the patient died about six hours after anaesthesia was started. The death was at least partly due to renal failure — in turn, the overwhelming effects of acidosis, hypercalcaemia and methaemoglobinuria. Presumptively, the large amounts of methaemoglobin molecules arriving in the glomerulus block the pores of the basement membrane causing anuria.

Just this year, it has become apparent that the genetic defect in malignant hyperthermia is on the gene for the calcium ion release channel of the sarcoplasmic reticulum. This raises the pleasant prospect of screening those about to undergo

ECF Ca²⁺

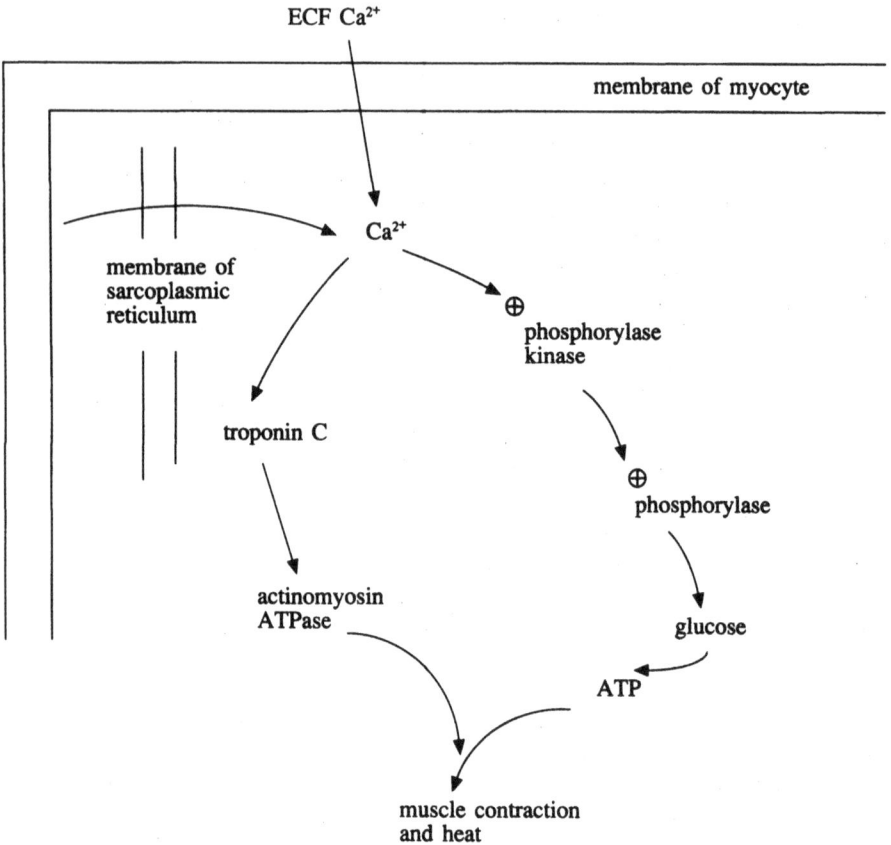

Fig. 35   Conceptual diagram of the role of calcium in malignant hyperthermia.

⊕ represents an activation step, whereas binding to troponin C results in a conformational change.

anaesthesia with DNA probes, since the present method (detecting contraction of a muscle biopsy in a caffeine solution) has not been judged reliable enough for general use, and of course requires a procedure under local anaesthesia to extract the tissue.

CALCIUM AND DEPRESSION

In April 1986, in the West Midlands of UK three members of a family (an elderly mother and her two adult sons) were shot and killed while asleep, and the 73-year-old husband and father was found seriously injured with head and facial wounds, which appeared to be self-inflicted. He died two weeks later. His medical history was reviewed and in 1982 he had been admitted to a district hospital for "biliary colic"; he had had low back pain, and was sweaty and shaking. He was given pethidine and subsequent radiology revealed gallstones which were treated by diet. Among the biochemical results at that time, the only abnormality on record was a total serum calcium of 2.75 mmol/l; this does seem very high, but on correction for serum albumin (Chap. 14b), it becomes 2.95 mmol/l.

At the inquest the surviving son said that he had noticed a steady deterioration in his father's mental well-being over the previous nine months, with apparent withdrawal and depression. The postmortem showed a grey nodule on the right lobe of the thyroid and minor focal nephrocalcinoisis.

Dr Acland who highlights the case (Ref. 3 below; we have presented it slightly differently in the interests of succinctness) feels that the deaths were all probably due to hypercalcaemia which as we saw above is often associated with depression. A single ionised calcium measurement at any time — remarked upon by the laboratory or the doctor reviewing the results — might have prevented the tragedy. Although this case relates to hyperparathyroidism in a sense, it is included here because it highlights a completely different facet of hypercalcaemia.

POINT

In the face of any mysterious metabolic crisis or even personality change, it is evidently worthwhile to measure serum calcium, preferably ionised calcium to avoid a messy correction for protein binding. Not all laboratories, even today, have the necessary ion-specific electrode technology, but — as the author of Ref. 1 below points out, in italics for emphasis, "Total calcium must give way to ionised calcium."

Further Reading

1. Kost GJ. The challenges of ionised calcium. *Arch Pathol Lab Med* **111** : 932–934, 1987.
2. Gronert GA, Mott J and Lee J. Aetiology of malignant hyperthermia. *Br J Anaes* **60** : 253–267, 1988.
3. Acland PR. Hypercalcaemia and depression. *Medicine Science and the Law* **28** : 139–142, 1988.
4. Wandrup J. Critical analytical and clinical aspects of ionised calcium in neonates. *Clin Chem* **35** : 2027–2033, 1989.

12b
Ions in Action

The importance of measuring the concentrations of certain ions — sometimes called electrolytes — in the body fluids becomes apparent to anybody on first encountering the biochemistry of disease. The crucial ions are sodium, potassium, chloride and bicarbonate — also calcium, but this is considered elsewhere (Chaps. 12a and 14b). Their measurement is central to the concept of homeostasis, the Bernardian hypothesis that it is the constancy of the milieu interieur which allows a free and independent life, so that it is thought best to keep them within narrow limits in the blood; however, some would say that the Bernardian principle has been taken too far, and that fluxes, as long as they are not catastrophic and unassociated with symptoms, may instead represent useful adaptation processes.

PASSING THE SALT

We have all read the chilling assertion that we are only bags of sea water — a dramatic oversimplification, of course, but nonetheless it is true that the main cation in our extracellular fluids is the same as in sea-water, namely sodium. Cells are active in pumping potassium into the cytoplasm and sodium to the exterior by means of the Na^+–K^+ ATPase pump. The function of sodium appears to be to maintain the osmotic pressure of the extracellular fluids, and therefore the extracellular volume, hence the blood pressure; whereas in the case of most physiologically active substances, it would be better to measure their concentrations inside cells, where they are exerting their biological activity, in respect of sodium we are intellectually justified in concentrating on its quantity in its natural habitat, i.e. serum.

Hyponatraemia is caused by:
(1) Water overload
(2) Congestive heart failure
(3) Diuretics
(4) Adrenal cortex insufficiency (e.g. Addison's disease)
(5) Syndrome of inappropriate secretion of antidiuretic hormone.

Hypernatraemia is generally due to:
(1) Dehydration
(2) Diabetes insipidus
(3) Hyperaldosteronism
(4) Salt overload and sodium containing drugs.

Some of these are purely concentration effects, dilutional in the case of water overload and congestive heart failure. The others represent loss or gain of body sodium mediated by drugs or hormones. However both hyper- and hyponatraemia are dangerous because they affect the volume of the brain, causing either swelling or dehydration according to the osmotic gradient, and therefore a disordered sensorium either way. Sudden changes appear to be the most dangerous, for there is generally an adaptation to less rapid fluxes. Hypernatraemia is rather uncommon — it is usually attributed to dehydration, and often in old people. Hyponatraemia on the other hand is a relatively common clinical finding. Consider the following:

PSEUD'S CORNER

A ten-year-old child, known to have been an insulin-dependent diabetic for some years previously, was brought into the emergency department because of abdominal pain and vomiting. At the same time, she was becoming progressively more drowsy, and indeed was comatose by the time she was seen by the medical officer. She was hypotonic and looked dehydrated, but the only other physical sign was the sheen of heavy chylomicronaemia in the vessels of the retina, so-called **lipaemia retinalis**. Some emergency clinical chemistry was ordered, and showed:

glucose	27.3	mmol/l	(reference interval, random specimen , 4–7.8)
sodium	93	mmol/l	(135–150)
potassium	3.1	mmol/l	(3.5–5.0)
chloride	63	mmol/l	(95–110)
bicarbonate	8.3	mmol/l	(22–31)
pH	7.13		
osmolality	415	mOsmol/kg	(275–300)

The medical officer obviously had to act fast; insulin was given both intramuscularly and intravenously to try to reduce the hyperglycaemia, as well as acidosis due to the (presumed) ketaemia. There was little improvement however, and in view of the very low serum electrolytes, a 0.9% saline infusion was started to try to raise them. However, when the child remained in the same comatose state, the consultant was called in. After going over the notes, he confirmed the lipaemia retinalis for himself, and immediately ordered that the saline drip be stopped. He also asked for blood lipids to be analysed as soon as possible (few laboratories, if any, will analyse cholesterol and triglycerides on a STAT basis.) When the report came back, with the child now a little improved, it indicated a staggering 23.1 mmol/l for total cholesterol (normally under 5 for a child of that age) and 193 mmol/l for triglycerides (usually under 1 mmol/l). He sent for a specimen of serum from the laboratory and passed it around — it was white, like milk.

The child had been exhibiting a pseudohyponatraemia, that is the sodium (and the other ions) only *seemed* low. This should have been suspected on two counts:

(1) The osmolality was not depressed, rather it was very high, and although no doubt the high figure was contributed to by the large amounts both of glucose and the presumed ketone bodies, sodium and chloride do remain the main contributors to osmolality.

(2) The hyperlipaemia observed in the retinal vessels should have been even more salutory.

Sodium and the other ions are dissolved only in the aqueous fraction of serum, but their concentration after analysis is traditionally expressed as mmol/l of whole serum, including the lipid compartment. Thus the denominator (volume) is artificially expanded and the concentrations of substances in the aqueous part seem low. The way round this problem is to centrifuge the serum to allow the fat to form a button at the top of the tube, the infranatant only to be analysed. Or alternatively, the laboratory can use an instrument with ion-specific electrodes for the potentiometric analysis of sodium and potassium. These instruments directly measure the activity (a thermodynamic concept, but almost the same as concentration) and so give a result independent of lipaemia. Sometimes a serum grossly loaded with protein, as in multiple myeloma, can be misleading in the same way.

So in this particular case the consultant fortunately intervened to avoid overloading the patient with sodium and risking potentially fatal depletion of water from the brain neurones.

POTASSIUM PROBLEMS

Drastic changes in potassium concentrations are generally acknowledged to be more dangerous than in the case of sodium, despite the fact that over 95% of the body potassium is inside the cells. Because the hydrogen ions in the circulation enter cells and are buffered, potassium is concomitantly expelled into the extracellular fluids, including the blood, to preserve electroneutrality. Thus acidosis is generally associated with hyperkalaemia.

Hyperkalaemia is also a result of:

(1) Congestive heart failure

(2) Acute and chronic renal failure

(3) Dehydration

(4) Muscle damage of all types, including malignant hyperthermia and heat stroke

(5) Adrenocortical insufficiency

Congestive heart failure causes potassium to accumulate in the blood as a result of metabolic acidosis and leakage of the ion from hypoxic cells. Muscle is a very large organ and if its cells are damaged, then comparatively enormous amounts of potassium may escape into the circulation, as in malignant hyperthermia (Chap. 12a).

Hypokalaemia is associated with:

(1) Diuretics (not the potassium sparing type)

(2) Vomiting and diarrhoea

(3) Impaired renal function

(4) Hypoaldosteronism (Conn's syndrome)

These obviously represent different ways in which potassium can be lost to the body.

One person with more than a passing interest in serum potassium is the anaesthetist, who habitually insists on a clinical chemistry panel for his patients before the induction. This is for a number of reasons: to act as a baseline for investigations after the operation; to screen for occult disorders; more immediately, to decide on whether anaesthetics may be safely given and if so, in which modalities. Potassium is important for all of these. Hypokalaemia causes cardiac arrhythmias and renal tubular nephropathy which would obviously be better avoided both during and after the operation. Measurement of serum potassium concentrations is especially important in patients taking digoxin since hypokalaemia may precipitate digoxin toxicity (nausea, vomiting, anorexia).

CHLORIDE

Chloride is usually thought of as a sort of adjunct to the other ions, falling in the blood when there is alkalosis due to bicarbonate accumulation (it has to fall to preserve electroneutrality), and rising in acidosis due to bicarbonate depletion from whatever reason (hyperchloraemic acidosis). However, it is essential to measure it, in its own right, for the calculation of anion gap (Chap. 13a) and serum osmolality which can be calculated (in mOsmol/kg when the components are expressed in mmol/l) as:

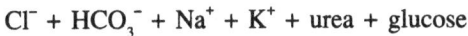

$$Cl^- + HCO_3^- + Na^+ + K^+ + urea + glucose$$

BICARBONATE

The other anion in serum which balances sodium and potassium is bicarbonate. In modern laboratories it is analysed in two ways: (i) in whole blood, as part of the blood gas panel; the measurement here is indirect, in that it is calculated using the

Henderson-Hasselbalch equation from pCO_2 and pH. Also (ii) it is analysed as carbon dioxide in serum. This needs some explanation — the analyser drives the equilibrium:

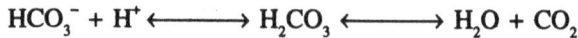

$$HCO_3^- + H^+ \longleftrightarrow H_2CO_3 \longleftrightarrow H_2O + CO_2$$

completely to the right by the addition of acid to the serum and then measures CO_2 by means of a specific electrode. But since the bicarbonate is always about twenty times greater than the other forms in the equilibrium above, the carbon dioxide as measured is an acceptable measure of that and it is in this light that the results is interpreted.

Coming back to a simplified version of the Henderson-Hasselbalch equation:

$$pH \propto bicarbonate \div pCO_2$$

it is obvious that the more bicarbonate there is in the blood, the higher will be its pH. In effect, excess bicarbonate produces a metabolic alkalosis; conversely carbon dioxide loading lowers the pH, giving a respiratory acidosis. Evidently a rise in both could leave the pH just about the same; this often happens in mixed acid-base disorders, e.g. a respiratory acidosis due to shock and a metabolic alkalosis due to vomiting.

Further Reading

1. Walmsley RN, Koay ESC and Watkinson LR. Acid-base disorders. Singapore University Press, pp. 219, 1989.
2. Swales JD. Dangers in treating hyponatraemia. *Br Med J* **294** : 261–262, 1987.
3. McCleane GJ. Preoperative investigations — the anaesthetists's perspective. *Br J Clin Pract* **44** : 5–8, 1990.

13a

The Old Acid

On all sides it is affirmed that medical students anathematise the topic of acid-base balance, and every textbook admits this to be true while declaring an intention to approach it in a truly digestible way. But the "antacid" attitude remains the problem, not the dyspepsia. Since here we are only writing notes, not comprehensive treatments of the various topics, we take the opportunity to show how one can acquire the skill to pick one's way through a problem of metabolic acidosis, and how interesting may be the clinical problem in itself.

Recall that, by definition, the main divisions into which acid-base disorders fall are:

Respiratory acidosis — high pCO_2
Respiratory alkalosis — low pCO_2
Metabolic acidosis — low bicarbonate
Metabolic alkalosis — high bicarbonate

In addition, there are the mixed types, which indeed may constitute the majority in most hospitals, when the pH may even be normal and which can be detected only by scrutiny of the bicarbonate, pCO_2 and pO_2. One generally has to consider three physiological systems, which swing into acid-base control one after the other: first of all, there is the almost instantaneous compensating effect of blood and intracellular buffers, then the respiratory centre in regulating the rate of breathing, with finally the kidneys responding somewhat later to eliminate acid or conserve bicarbonate.

METABOLIC INVESTIGATION

An old man in a comatose condition is brought into the emergency room by his relatives. He had been seen working round the house, and was found unconscious in the garden shed some hours later. There is no smell of alcohol on the breath, nor any sign of injury, and no marks of burning round the mouth or pharynx. Of course you suspect a heart attack, or perhaps poisoning, so after the initial physical examination some STAT chemistry is called for, hopefully with the results back within about 20 minutes after you first see the patient. At the same time the bladder is cannulated to obtain enough urine for a toxicology screen. These first results are as follows:

respiratory rate	28/min	pulse	120/min	
bp	116/70	temp	37°C	
pH (arterial)	6.98	pCO_2	15 mm Hg	(normal 35–45)
creatine kinase	40 U/l	bicarbonate	5 mmol/l	(22–31)
	(60–370)			

The patient is therefore unlikely to have a had a coronary (although care should be exercised here because creatine kinase needs time to rise if this is what has happened, see Chap. 6a) but obviously the old man is very acidotic. This is in concert with the rapid respiratory rate as the lungs attempt to blow off acid, represented in the gaseous phase by carbon dioxide. It is a metabolic acidosis, and bicarbonate is quickly infused to try to bring the pH up, while the second group of results from the laboratory are awaited. Meanwhile the various causes of metabolic acidosis are kept in mind.

(1) Diabetic ketoacidosis
(2) Lactic acidosis (hypoxia, shock)
(3) Salicylate ingestion
(4) Methanol, ethylene or propylene glycol poisoning
(5) Ingestion of mineral acids
(6) Diarrhoea.

The relatives say that the old man is not diabetic, and had not had diarrhoea. So it begins to look even more likely that he had taken some obnoxious substance. The second batch of results give:

sodium	144	mmol/l	(reference interval, 135–150)
chloride	108	mmol/l	(95–105)
potassium	4.8	mmol/l	(3.5–5)
urea	9.5	mmol/l	(3.2–7.5)
creatinine	190	μmol/l	(70–133)
glucose	4.6	mmol/l	(random, 4–7.8)

So the acidosis is of the high anion gap type, that is

$$(K^+ + Na^+) - (Cl^- + HCO_3^-) = 37 \text{ (normal 12–20)}$$

Quickly a serum lactate is requested, and proves to be 7.3 mmol/l, so it probably partly explains the high ion gap. The condition is now even more unlikely to be due to diabetic ketoacidosis, and in any case the glucose is normal. Meanwhile, the results of the urine screen come back and prove negative for drugs of abuse, salicylate, methanol and ethanol. But there are some suspicious crystals which the laboratory says "may" be calcium oxalate. You now have the diagnosis, for the product of the metabolism of ethylene glycol, which is often kept in old bottles in garages and sheds, is oxalic acid. This avidly forms a salt with calcium which tends to precipitate in the kidney (Fig. 36).

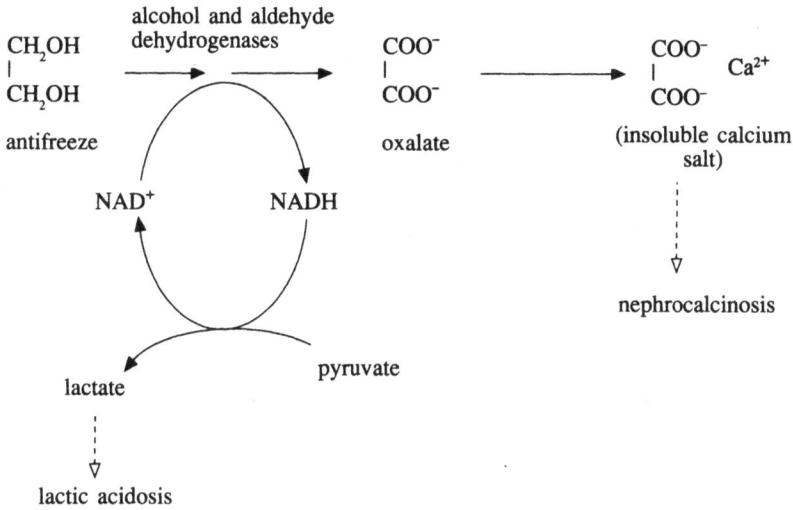

Fig. 36 The metabolism of ethylene glycol.

In this instance the chemical formulae are helpful for an understanding of the process.

The patient is carefully titrated back to pH 7.4, and an injection of ethanol in saline is administered. This competes with the alcohol dehydrogenase which is catalysing the production of the noxious and nephrotoxic oxalate. But if the dose of the poison appears to have been a massive one, then forced diuresis or dialysis will be necessary. There is no simple test for ethylene glycol in the blood, but it could later be estimated by high pressure liquid chromatography if necessary. It would be highly desirable to store a specimen of blood against that necessity.

If the patient recovers, then his kidney function will be have to be assessed carefully, for there is already suspicion that the deposition of calcium oxalate in the tubules has caused a rising urea and creatinine, as seen above. We may also find out how he came to ingest it, whether from a mislabelled bottle in the garage, or deliberately.

THE RESULTS COME OUT THE SAME

Dr Eva Lester has provided a somewhat macabre anecdote about blood pH. Her laboratory staff repeated an arterial blood gas determination not once, but several times and the results still looked bizarre. She pulled out the previous results for the same patient (done 20 minutes before) and compared them. They were as below:

	First sampling	Second sampling	Reference intervals	
pH	6.73	7.29	7.35–7.45	
PCO_2	66	151	35–45	mm Hg
HCO_3^-	9	72	22–31	mmol/l
pO_2	65	23	75–100	mm Hg

The first results indicate a very severe respiratory and metabolic acidosis. The low pO_2 indicates that respiration is very poor. Dr Lester notes that when she saw the second set, she knew immediately that the patient had been dead when the blood was taken. Adapting the Henderson-Hasselbalch approximation again (see last Chap. 12):

$$pH \quad \propto \quad \frac{HCO_3^-}{pCO_2} \quad or \quad \frac{9}{66} \quad and \quad \frac{72}{151}$$

(first sampling)   (second sampling)

One can see now why the pH appeared to normalise with the second sampling. With breathing stopped and a certain amount of anaerobic metabolism still taking place, the carbon dioxide rose steeply, enough to generate appreciable bicarbonate at the same time. However, the values produced by the blood gas analyser are themselves incompatible with life. Dr Lester deprecates sending pseudo-autopsy samples to the laboratory but acknowledges the pressure on the medical staff to deny the fact of death.

Further Reading

1. Buckley, BM. Metabolic effects of poisoning. *Med Int* No 61 : 2504–2507, 1989.

13b

Erythropoietin for Well-Being

The patient with chronic renal failure is subject to multiple fluid and electrolyte disturbances, protein wasting, hypertension, neuropathies and convulsions. The introduction of kidney transplants and dialysis has greatly improved prospects in these dire circumstances, but in respect of the former, the publicity given to the unfortunate cases of organ peddling has highlighted the worldwide shortage of donors, and the latter has its own hazards (Chap. 18d). A further and severe manifestation of kidney disease is anaemia. In a survey by the European Dialysis and Transplant Association, 18% of dialysis patients were found to be so anaemic as to be dependent on regular blood transfusions. The reason for the anaemia can be traced to the protein erythropoietin, which was discovered as long ago as the first decade of this century. It is largely produced by the juxtatubular cells of the kidney — only 10–20% is derived from an alternative source, the liver. It is synthesised with one more amino acid than the active, circulating form, an idiosyncracy, for although many hormones are synthesised in a precursor form (see for example proinsulin), the final processing usually involves removal of a fairly substantial peptide moiety. Erythropoietin is released in response to hypoxia, as can be demonstrated by its increment in the blood of subjects moving to high altitudes, or in patients with haemoglobinopathies like thalassaemia — and commits undifferentiated erythroid precursors in the bone marrow to development into erythrocytes. A classic feedback cycle operates — hypoxia results in the synthesis of erythropoietin, possibly through the mediation of a sensor haemoprotein, and when oxygen tension is restored, the production of the stimulating factor is switched off again.

One of the ways the kidney was established to be the main source of erythropoietin was the demonstration of a 200-fold increase of mRNA after anaemia induction — this also shows that erythropoietin is not released from preformed granules but is synthesised *de novo* by the hypoxic stimulus.

The haemopoietic system is thus both finely modulated and extremely active — the average adult generates 2.4 million red blood cells **per second**, or half a metric tonne of them over a lifetime. The precariousness of the system, too, is demonstrated by patients who have had kidney transplantation and who develop erythrocytosis, that is an elevation in the red cell mass, with a normal plasma volume. This is generally considered to be due to abnormally high production of erythropoietin as a result of defective feedback regulation of production by the remaining native kidney.

An obvious response to the anaemia of renal failure is to administer erythropoietin, if it can be obtained. Preparation of therapeutic quantities from natural sources — say animal blood — would be near to impossible. Once again however, recombinant DNA technology offered a way out of the difficulty.

HUMAN RECOMBINANT ERYTHROPOIETIN

The biochemical contribution to the success of erythropoietin therapy was its initial purification and sequencing, the cloning of the gene for it, and the harvesting and purification of the gene product. Erythropoietin is a molecule of 39 000 molecular weight, that is, 165 amino acids, but the molecule as a whole bears 40% carbohydrate, principally sialic acid. The recombinant product from *E coli* consists of the naked protein, which however is just as biologically active. It is thought that the advantage of the native glycoprotein form may be its relative potection against over-rapid degradation by the liver. The gene sequence is highly conserved among species, attesting to the importance of the protein products for survival.

Recombinant erythropoietin may be given intravenously but recent studies have indicated that the subcutaneous route may allow a lower dosage schedule. Its efficacy is shown by a rise in haematocrit and in red blood cell count (it has no effect on leukocytes) and — related to the enhanced oxygenation of tissues — the patients, taken as a group, show fewer depressive episodes, but increased exercise tolerance, resistance to fatigue, cognitive function, libido, and general well-being. A spin-off, unrelated to the condition of the patient per se, is the enormous saving in the number of units required from blood banks.

As usual there are snags, among them a thrombotic tendency, flu-like symptoms, hypertension, hyperkalaemia and seizures, but most authorities indicate that these are outweighed by the benefits enumerated above. In any case, it is thought that such complications may be avoided by increasing the dose of erythropoietin gradually.

Another perhaps tangential problem is that the enhanced haemopoiesis causes an extra demand for iron, so if haemoglobin does not rise as expected after treatment with erythropoietin, then iron deficiency may be the cause.

TESTING FOR IRON DEFICIENCY

It might be thought, reasonably enough, that the way to assess for a deficit of iron in patients receiving erythropoietin, and in others, is to measure the concentration of the metal in the serum. Unfortunately, serum iron can be affected not only by iron nutrition but by a host of other factors, for example time of day (it has an immense diurnal variation) and the presence of acute or chronic infection (even a slight common cold will reduce it). An alternative which may be measured is transferrin, the iron transporting protein of serum, which is synthesised in increased quantities in iron deficiency; in fact it corresponds to the old total iron binding capacity or TIBC. However, it is also a negative acute phase protein — it decreases in inflammation or malignancy. It also tends to be reduced in malnutrition, chronic liver disease and nephrotic syndrome. In other words, like serum iron it is just too labile to interpret with confidence. The other iron storage protein, ferritin, the bulk of which is in the liver but which appears in small quantities in the circulation, is now considered to be the best index of iron deficiency, in which it is decreased. It is not free from positive (rather than negative, as for tranferrin) acute phase responses, but these can generally be taken into account in the interpretation. It can now be measured readily by immunoassay, so the response of patients receiving erythropoietin will no doubt be assessed by full blood counts and ferritin determinations at regular intervals.

OTHER USES OF ERYTHROPOIETIN

Erythropoietin can be used to boost the number of red cells in the circulation in advance of autologous transfusion — the practice of banking one's own blood prior to a scheduled surgical operation, or even on the off-chance of one — to avoid the possible hazards of cross matching, and unknown viruses and prions in donor blood (although AIDS and hepatitis B at least should be eliminated by modern screening methods unless you are unlucky enough to have a donor who has been infected but who has not yet produced sufficient titre of antibody.)

Erythropoietin can be used to stimulate transplanted bone marrow. In AIDS patients, chemotherapy with zidovudine is liable to cause anaemia and erythropoietin has aroused much interest as a rescue agent. Finally, many premature babies appear to have low levels of it and administration of the recombinant form is thought likely to promote differentiation of the erythroid precursors.

But further, as we mention later in the case of growth hormone (Chap. 14a), the potential benefits of erythropoietin have not gone unnoticed by unscrupulous athletics coaches and managers, who perceive that they could induce a superior oxygen loading capacity into their charges by slipping it into the cocktail of substances they inject already. Since it is a natural substance of varying concentration in the blood of any one individual, it is extremely difficult to prove that it is of exogenous origin in an athlete, although there may be a way round this by measuring the amount of sialic acid attached to the erythropoietin molecule in suspect blood. As noted above, the pharmacological, recombinant form is non-glycated. But such manoeuvres and counter-manoeuvres are only just being developed.

Comment

About ten human haemopoietic growth factors are now known, all glycoproteins of moderate size. Surprisingly though, the associated carbohydrate is not involved in biological activity of any of them as so far determined. Other than erythropoietin, these substances consist of the so-called colony stimulating factors and certain of the interleukins (Chap. 17b). The interactions among the group are complex and will be a matter for the specialist for some time to come. They will probably all be used as drugs at some time in the future, but for now erythropoietin holds centre stage.

Further Reading

1. Anon. Erythropoietin reaches the pharmacy. *Lancet* ii : 1245–1246, 1989.
2. Hambley H and Ghulam GJ. Erythropoietin: an old friend revisited. *Br Med J* **300** : 621–622, 1990.

14a

Is Smaller Worse?

"While it seems desirable to prevent the avoidable occurrence of a group of Lilliputians, it is quite another matter to stimulate the existence of a population of Brobdignagians."

— Dr I Gunn in a gloss on Gulliver's Travels

You will recognise, in the title, the inverse of the first reference below wherein the author more or less answers his question by remarking that one need only reflect on the expectations commonly encountered in male-female bonding, in that men are expected to pair up with women shorter than themselves, and it is considered a matter of comment when a small man like Dudley Moore marries a tall woman like Susan Anton.

Growth during the prenatal period and the first year of life depends on nutrition. This is illustrated by the babies of diabetic mothers, whose large size is due to the continuous surfeit of glucose available to them after conception. In childhood however the rate is determined by the secretion of growth hormone, vagaries of which cause the extremes of pituitary dwarfism on the one hand, and acromegaly/giantism on the other. Growth hormone (otherwise known as somatotrophin, STH) is secreted by the anterior pituitary in the form of a 191 amino acid single chain monomer stabilised by two disulphide cross-links. Its sequence has some homology with prolactin although the importance of any cross-activity is uncertain in humans.

In tissues, growth hormone has a dichotomous effect (Fig. 37). Its growth-promoting activities in cartilage and muscle are mediated through a class of peptides called somatomedins, or insulin-like growth factors (IGFs) since they have homologies with proinsulin. IGF-1 (somatomedin C) is the best known of the group and at the present time may be routinely assayed in the hospital laboratory. IGFs are probably largely synthesised in the liver, and interact with receptors in such tissues as manifest lateral and longtitudinal growth. In liver and adipose tissue there are receptors for the parent hormone itself, and in these tissues it is largely antagonistic to insulin. Fig. 37 is a reminder that that there may be lesions at any point in the whole sequence: thus, there may be failure of secretion of the releasing factor, or of growth hormone itself, or of IGF-1, and there may be defects in any of the range of receptors from the pituitary to the target tissues. Pinpointing the exact site of a problem along such an axis is of course common to much of endocrinological investigation.

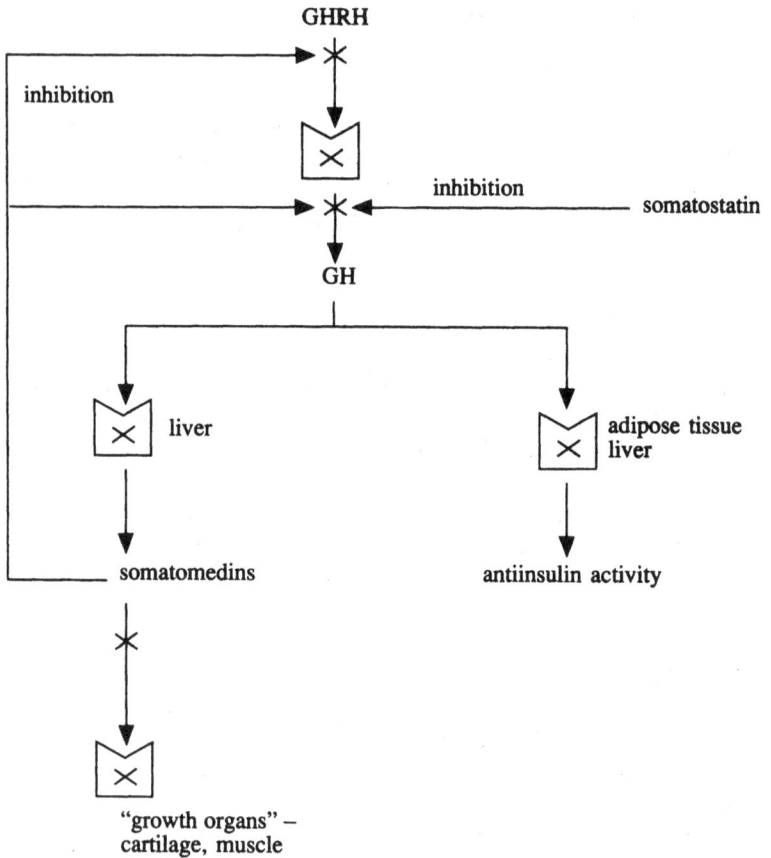

Fig. 37 The growth hormone-somatomedin axis.

A block designated by ✕ theoretically could occur at any point where there is a receptor ⊔ or where the sequence depends on synthesis of functional protein.

GROWTH PROBLEMS

Growth charts sit on doctors' desks so that they can distinguish, in a reasonably objective way, true growth problems from the mere impressions of worried parents. One recommendation is to investigate immediately any child who is growing at less than the third centile velocity — in other words, at a rate less than 97% of the whole population. In the first instance, more general possible reasons for the retardation are investigated, e.g. malnutrition, chronic infections, malabsorption, respiratory disease, thalassaemia, hypothyroidism and kidney disease. A lack of energy or of its utilisation can be rationalised as the reason for growth failure in all of these except the last — in chronic renal failure, which is not reversed by dialysis, it may possibly be due to the unremitting acidosis or mineral depletion, or both. It is also maintained by some that social and emotional deprivation can in itself cause growth retardation. If no other cause can be found, then there is the presumption that a failure somewhere along the effector pathway for growth hormone is responsible.

TESTING FOR GROWTH HORMONE

In the basal state, the secretion of growth hormone is episodic, and even in normal persons it may not be detectable in the serum over several blood samplings, so some sort of stimulus is required to show that the cells of the pituitary are competent to release the hormone. There are two approaches, physiological and pharmacological. Into the first category come exercise and sleep, for both stimulate release of the hormone. Apart from the taking of blood, these cause little distress, and no danger, to the patient.

Pharmacological tests are as follows: the hypotensive agent clonidine, a β-adrenergic blocker reducing sympathetic nerve outflow, stimulates growth hormone secretion and can be given orally. Arginine, for reasons which are not entirely clear, also stimulates growth hormone secretion — it is infused over thirty minutes and a peak of hormone secretion should occur shortly after that. Insulin-induced hypoglycaemia is the easiest of the pharmacological tests to understand in terms of classical endocrinology. Growth hormone being an antagonist to insulin, is secreted in response to a rapidly falling blood glucose. If the hypothalamic-pituitary axis is patent in this respect, then the resulting surge of hormone can be measured. As the test progresses, blood glucose must be monitored and only when it reaches less than 2 mmol/l is it worthwhile to proceed to take frequent blood samples for growth hormone measurements. If it drops precipitously below 2 mmol/l, the test has to be aborted immediately and the dextrose infusion kept at hand administered. Usually cortisol is assayed at the same time, since it is also an insulin antagonist and its rise will be another index of pituitary function. There is a characteristic pattern of response in growth hormone secreting deficiency, as opposed to normals (Fig. 38).

Many authorities like to do a physiological test, and if this is indecisive, proceed to one of the pharmacological ones. Each of them, however, can do no more than demonstrate a preformed, releasable pool of growth hormone in the pituitary at the time the challenge is applied; if there has been a pulse of the hormone recently, for whatever cause, and the gland is empty, then the response will be lacking. A high baseline value with a negative response may be a clue to this situation.

IgF-1 can be assayed to test the integrity of the pathway distal to reaction of growth hormone with receptors on liver but at the present time, assessment of the various receptors is a difficult task. However, a challenge test can be done with growth hormone releasing hormone to see whether any defect resides in the hypothalamus.

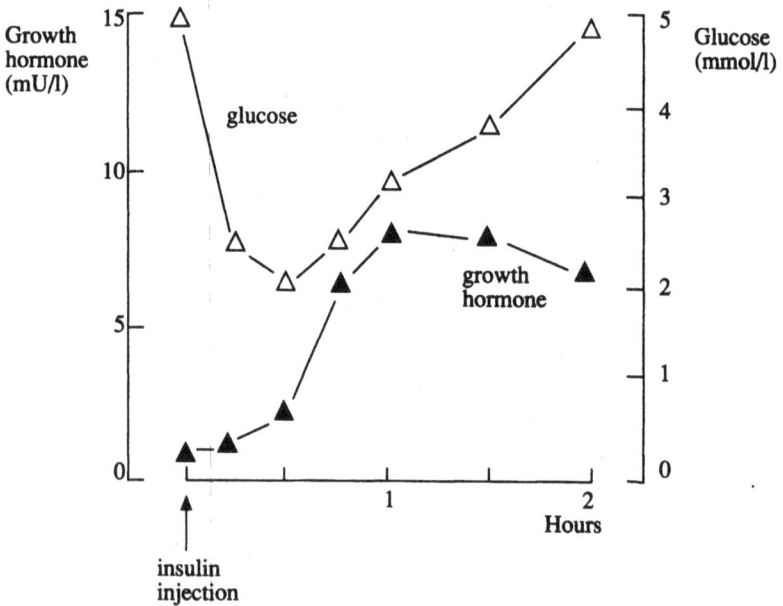

Fig. 38 The insulin hypoglycaemia test.

The normal response of serum glucose and growth hormone to the administration of insulin is shown. In the absence of a patent secretion of growth hormone the lower curve is flattened.

THE NEW GROWTH HORMONE

One can well imagine the problems, in the days before biochemical engineering, of acquiring and processing sufficient human pituitaries to obtain useable amounts of growth hormone, not to mention the purification of the product to standards commensurate with safety. Indeed this last was never achieved, since some preparations retained the agent for Jacob-Creutzfeldt disease, the presumed prion (Chap. 1d). When the engineers set out to produce the hormone from a non-pathogenic strain of *E. coli* they found it easier to make an initial product with short basic peptide attached at the amino-terminal end. This could be selectively retained on a chromatographic column following which most of the unwanted contaminants were washed off. This peptide was subsequently removed with an enzyme, an aminopeptidase, to give a product identical to human pituitary-derived growth hormone.

A SHOT IN THE ARM FOR THE ELDERLY

When recombinant growth hormone became available, despite its high cost, trials were mounted on all sorts of people. You cannot give a protein-like growth hormone (and insulin) by mouth, of course, so volunteers had to be injected intramuscularly. Since it was known that growth hormone secretion gradually declines with age, one such trial involved men of 60–81 years. Part of the impetus was that the decline in growth hormone secretion seems to be correlated with increasing adiposity and decreasing muscle mass. Growth hormone did indeed reverse both these trends. It also increased vertebral bone density, exercise capacity, isometric strength, and metabolic rate in another trial on men and women with established growth hormone deficiency. Fasting serum glucose rose in all groups — herein lies the problem, in that growth hormone is potentially diabetogenic. In animals, it has also been established to cause arthralgia, arthritis, hypertension, oedema and congestive heart failure.

The ethical isues of growth hormone administration to the apparently normal are being hotly debated. It seems reasonably certain, however, that practitioners in the next few years, especially as the price of recombinant growth hormone falls (a full course is currently about US $14 000 per year) will have requests from elderly patients seeking shots of it to obtain at least some of the components of rejuvenation. Requests may also come from athletes seeking an enhanced lean body mass — indeed this is already happening covertly. Of course unlike synthetic drugs (Chap. 5b) but like erythropoetin (Chap. 13b), it will be difficult for regulatory bodies to detect abuse, or even establish that the concept of abuse is applicable. All medical authorities are adamant that treating normal healthy children with growth hormone to increase their strengths or statures (to enable them to be recruited into elite guards regiments, or join basketball teams, for example) is inadmissible because we do not know enough about the long-term effects of the preparations now available.

AUTOCANNIBALISM AND GROWTH HORMONE

Research needs rather to be directed to the possibility that synthetic growth hormone may be efficacious in severe catabolic illnesses, like post-surgical marasmus, burn injury, sepsis and renal failure. As long ago as the 1930s, Cuthbertson showed that even minor trauma is followed by a general catabolism of body protein — in itself no doubt a survival mechanism, providing amino acids for conversion to glucose by gluconeogenesis and perhaps for the synthesis of acute phase proteins in the liver. However, hypercatabolism ("autocannibalism") appears to affect immune function and it would very desirable were it not allowed to proceed too far.

Trials using growth hormone at about five times the dose used for growth hormone deficiency itself have been mounted. One of them appeared to indicate a shortened period in hospital for severely burned children.

In summary, you may end up prescribing bioengineered growth hormone for a lot of different people in the long run.

Further Reading

1. Diekema DS. Is taller really better? Growth hormone therapy in short children. *Perspectives in Biology and Medicine* **34** : 109–121, 1990.
2. Brook C and Hindmarsh PC. Tests for growth hormone secretion. *Arch Dis Childhood* **66** : 85–87, 1991.
3. Vance ML. Growth hormone for the elderly. *N Eng J Med* **323** : 52–54, 1990.
4. Ross RJM, Miell JP and Buchanan CR. Avoiding autocannibalism. *Br Med J* **303** : 1147–1148, 1991.

14b

Bones, Groans, Moans and Stones

Hypercalcaemia is a common feature of patients with carcinomas, and it can precipitate a wide variety of symptoms such as anorexia, vomiting, constipation, thirst, abdominal pain and urinary tract stone formation. Because of the non-specific nature of these symptoms, they can easily be ascribed to a whole range of spurious causes, and it is important to measure calcium levels in cancer patients at frequent intervals.

Excluding the haematological malignancies, there are two main clinical groups of malignancy-associated hypercalcaemia.

(1) Those involving bony metastatic deposits. (The classical five tumours that metastasise to bone are breast, lung, prostate, kidney and thyroid.)
   There is resulting calcium release from the area of the metastasis. The exact biochemical mechanisms at the basis of this are not really clear. One suggestion is that prostaglandins, especially E_2, may be mediators as they are known to be powerful bone resorbing factors. Other possible factors are the cytokines, especially tumour necrosis factor and interleukin-1 (Chap. 17b) which have also been shown to have the capacity to initiate bone resorption. Whatever the mechanism, bony metastatic deposits are a common cause of hypercalcaemia.

(2) The humoral hypercalcaemia of malignancy syndrome (HHMS).
   Older medical textbooks refer to "ectopic parathyroid hormone syndrome of malignancy"; the newer term implies less certainty about the nature of the condition, but is no improvement in terms of length or pronounceability.

HUMORAL CALCAEMIA OF MALIGNANCY

The result of parathyroid hormone secretion is bone resorption and but it also acts upon the kidney to reduce calcium excretion and conversely increase excretion of phosphate and cAMP, the combination of these actions resulting in a raising of plasma calcium and a decrease in plasma phosphate. Indeed, this is the pattern observed in HHMS. Some of the earlier work using radioimmunoassay indicated that plasma parathyroid hormone was raised in a group of patients with bronchogenic carcinoma, but with increasing sophistication in the technique over the years it became apparent that authentic hormone was not identical to the immunoreactive species observed in these groups of cancer patients. Thus the hypercalcaemic factor of malignancy is due to a parathyroid hormone-like substance, not the intact hormone itself. In addition, in these patients plasma chloride concentrations were low and bicarbonate high, the converse to the situation usually found in primary hyperparathyroidism where the intact hormone has a profound effect on the kidneys. (This of course is a hyperchloraemic acidosis, a form of metabolic acidosis with a normal anion gap.)

In summary, there is evidence that in some patients with HHMS, in which no or minimal bony metastases are present, a protein with parathyroid-like activity is circulating. Studies have now confirmed that this protein can activate adenylate cyclase of kidney membranes to increase cAMP production in a manner similar to the native hormone, but it has a diverse antigenic activity.

Purification techniques and sequencing studies have shown extensive homology with parathyroid hormone around the amino-terminal end but differences elsewhere in the molecule. It was concluded that the protein probably arose from the parathyroid hormone gene by duplication, but now remains a distinct gene product. The similarity at the amino-terminal end does explain its binding cell receptors for the native hormone.

It is important to note that the parathyroid-like protein has also been found to be produced by normal epithelial cells and the human skin cells called keratinocytes, suggesting a possible physiological role. There are also some preliminary data to suggest that it may be involved in calcium regulation fetus transport and may also have a role in lactation.

This parathyroid-related protein, as it is now generally called, has been shown to be also produced by some squamous cell bronchial carcinomas and also by some breast carcinomas. Its similarity to PTH would account in part for the increased urinary phosphate excretion and hypercalcaemia seen in these conditions.

PRACTICAL POINTS

Hypercalcaemia is a relatively common clinical condition particularly, as we have noted above, in patients with certain carcinomas. Because of the vague, non-specific symptoms of hypercalcaemia, it is very useful to measure the serum calcium concentrations in such groups. As about 50% of calcium in the blood is protein-bound, principally to albumin (the most abundant plasma protein at a concentration of about 40 g/l), serum calcium concentrations should ideally be corrected for the albumin. One such proposed correction is

Corrected calcium = calcium as + (40 − albumin) × 0.02
(mmol/l)   measured   (g/l)
                     (mmol/l)

So a low plasma or serum calcium value in the presence of a low albumin, when corrected, may give a "normal" value. Therefore, always ask to see the serum albumin when interpreting calcium results, otherwise dramatic errors in clinical decision making may result. Or, ask the laboratory to measure ionised calcium (Chap 12a). How does all this work out in practice?

A 67-years-old retired mechanic presented to the local hospital with dyspnoea, haemoptysis (coughing blood) and weight loss. A chest X-ray revealed a "shadow" in the left upper zone of his lung, which was shown to be a squamous cell carcinoma when the biopsy taken by bronchoscopy was studied by the pathologist. The tumour was considered to be inoperable and a course of radiotherapy was commenced with some regression of the lesion and symptomatic improvement over the following months. A year later, the patient was admitted to the casualty department of the same hospital complaining of abdominal pain, vomiting, polyuria, polydipsia and weakness. Blood was taken for emergency analysis, and sent to the biochemistry laboratory. The results were:

sodium	152	mmol/l	(reference interval, 135–150)
potassium	3.0	mmol/l	(3.5–5)
albumin	46	g/l	(39–50)
calcium	3.97	mmol/l	(2.10–2.6)
urea	8.6	mmol/l	(3.2–7.5)
glucose	3.9	mmol/l	(4–7.8, random)
phosphate	0.5	mmol/l	(0.8–1.4)

The hypernatraemia and moderately raised urea indicate a degree of dehydration consistent with the polyuria and vomiting which the patient himself reported. The hypokalaemia is probably also the result of the vomiting. The polydipsia and polyuria make an initial consideration of diabetes necessary, but the glucose is normal if not low for a random specimen.

It is the calcium and phosphate with which we are most concerned. The former looks very high but cannily, we correct it for the albumin concentration, achieving a revised figure, *per* the formula above, of 3.85 — still a massive increment over normal. The hypophosphataemia tends to confirm HHMS in a patient with a known malignancy. The results unfortunately indicate that the original tumour had metastasised and the patient was urgently referred to the oncologist who after a number of other tests (haematology, bone scans) was able to suggest only palliative treatment.

Further Reading

1. Kemp BE. Humoral hypercalcaemia of malignancy. *Aust N Z J Med* **18** : 287–295, 1988.
2. Ralston SH, Gallacher SJ, Patel U, et al. Cancer-associated hypercalcaemia. *Ann Intern Med* **112** : 499–504, 1991.

14c

The Thyroid: At Threes and Fours

"I once believed that with increasing experience as a thyroidologist I would be able to sharpen my clinical diagnostic acumen progressively and to diagnose ever more subtle types of incipient thyroid dysfunction. I concentrated mightily on the skin, the distribution of lateral eyebrow hair, and the speed of tendon reflex return ... but ... technology has finally brought thyroidologists to their knees."
— Dr Colum A Gorman

To what extent can clinicians still rely upon physical signs to diagnose thyroid disease, and to what extent does the clinical chemistry laboratory have something better to offer? Let us first revise some of the basic biochemistry of the thyroid gland. The thyroid secretes two principle hormones (three if we include calcitonin).

Thyroxine (T4) exists in the free form in serum only to the extent of 0.02%, the rest being protein bound, mainly to thyroxine binding globulin (TBG), but also to albumin and prealbumin. This recalls the important concept of "free" hormones, the physiologically active forms, as opposed to the totals which reflect protein bound hormone as well. Thus laboratories now habitually measure free hormone concentrations as opposed to totals which might be confounded by variations in serum TBG (which is raised, for example, in pregnancy and oral contraceptive use).

Albumin and prealbumin are equally likely to vary independently of thyroid status.

Triiodothyronine (T3) exists in the serum in concentrations about one hundred times lower than those of T4; however, about 0.36% of the T3 is found in the free form. About 80% of the actions of thyroid hormones are thought to be due to free T3 and only 20% by free T4. Furthermore, about 80% of serum T3 is thought to be derived from peripheral conversion of T4 with the remainder being derived directly from the thyroid gland.

ACTIONS OF THYROID HORMONES

It is worth remembering these actions as they help to explain some of the symptoms that patients with florid thyroid abnormalities may present with.

(1) They are essential for normal growth and development. Hence children with thyroid deficiency often show growth retardation and impaired brain development.

(2) They cause an increase in basal metabolic rate. Thus patients with thyroid hormone deficiency tend to become overweight and lethargic and tend to dislike cold weather. Conversely, patients with hyperthyroidism tend to lose weight, incline to sweatiness, and dislike hot weather.

(3) T4 and T3 can increase the sensitivity of tissues to catecholamines, which may partly explain why patients with myxoedema, that is thyroid underactivity, have a slow pulse rate, whereas the converse is true in hyperthyroid states.

THYROID STIMULATING HORMONE

The thyroid, like many other endocrine glands, is under the influence of the pituitary. Thyroid stimulating hormone (TSH) is released from the anterior pituitary, itself under the releasing action of thyroid releasing hormone (TRH) secreted from the hypothalamus. TSH acts upon the thyroid gland and ultimately causes the increased secretion of T4. Feedback control from circulating plasma thyroid hormones regulates the TSH release from the pituitary gland, so it is high and low in hypo- and hyperthyroidism, respectively. Since it is evidently a nuisance to measure very small amounts of free T4 and/or T3, or allowing for their binding to proteins in measuring totals, it occurred to clinicians a long time ago that a straight measurement of TSH might be more useful and convenient. Reinforcing the idea is that TSH represents an amplification system, that is typically TSH changes tenfold in comparison to free T4. This is fine for the detection of hypothyroidism, but in hyperthyroidism where TSH secretion is suppressed, methods have to be developed to detect very low amounts of it. Put more scientifically, you have to distinguish with statistical confidence the lower limit of normal (about 0.5 mU/l) from a concentration defined as hyperthyroid. This means that TSH estimations of high detectability, or "sensitive" TSH methods as they are called, must quantitate concentrations around 0.1 mU/l. Immunometric assays can now achieve this.

COMMON CAUSES OF HYPOTHYROIDISM

Primary hypothyroidism
 (1) Autoimmune disease, e.g. Hashimoto's disease
 (2) Thyroid gland damage, e.g. surgery or radiation
 (3) Iodine deficiency
 (4) Dyshormonogenesis, i.e. abnormality of thyroid hormone synthesis.
Secondary Hypothyroidism
 (1) Pituitary disease.

COMMON CAUSES OF HYPERTHYROIDISM

 (1) Graves' disease (thyroid stimulated by immunoglobins)
 (2) Toxic adenoma or multinodular goitre
 (3) Overtreatment with thyroxine (T4).

THE STRATEGY OF TESTING FOR THYROID DISORDERS

As the quotation at the head implies, detection of thyroid dysfunction has evolved from observing the constellation of physical signs to scanning the asterixes on the radioimmunoassay printout. This is so especially for the occult forms and — very importantly — for neonatal screening. The question is, What should be the choice of tests? Or rather, which should be the single first line test — remember that doing multiple testing increases predictive value but at the same time escalates the expense.

   With development of TSH estimations of high detectability, clinicians have gradually come to accept it as the first line test of choice. In primary hypothyroidism, i.e. the result of some sort of insult to the thyroid gland itself, the TSH is raised (in an attempt to stimulate the thyroid gland) and T4 and T3 are reduced, as would be expected. It is more unusual for hypothyroidism to be due to anterior pituitary disease (secondary hypothyroidism), when TSH and free T4 and T3 are all reduced. Inhibitory autoantibodies to thyroid components in the serum can be measured later to facilitate the diagnosis of autoimmune hypothyroidism, if this is suspected. In hyperthyroidism, serum TSH is invariably suppressed and serum free T4 and T3 are increased.

Even when thyroid deficiency and overactivity are detected, of course, the differential diagnosis is yet to come, *qua* the listing above. And there are the usual snags involving rare diseases. For example there is the rare condition called T3 thyrotoxicosis where only free T3 is elevated and not T4.

A SLIGHT CASE OF PHARMACOPHOBIA

A 68-year-old man with a history of hyperthyroidism due to Graves' disease, treated by total thyroidectomy, was seen for follow-up at medical outpatients. He had been placed on thyroxine at 150 μg/day as replacement therapy. When seen, he stated that he was "on top of the world" but the doctor, upon physical examination, noticed slow relaxing ankle jerks (a useful sign of hypothyroidism) and the old man said that he had put on weight since the operation. The doctor therefore took blood for thyroid function testing. He was surprised a few days later to receive the following results:

TSH   14   mU/l   (reference interval, 0.5–4.0)
Free T4   36   pmol/l   (10–25)

He phoned the laboratory tactfully suggesting that it might be in error, not being able to rationalize the elevated T4 and TSH in conjunction. (It could occur in secondary hyperthyroidism, but what are the chances of a Graves patient subsequently developing a TSH secreting pituitary tumour?)

However, the chemical pathologist did have a suggestion — could the the patient in a fit of conscience have taken his medication just before reporting to the surgery? The elevated TSH would then reflect a hypothyroid state, the elevated T4 the recent oral intake. The doctor had another look at the patient and noticed in addition the dry skin, and though he did not accuse the old man directly of the small deceit, he elicted the fact that he was constipated and needed the heating in his house turned up high. It all fitted the picture of a progressive hypothyroidism — what then could be done but deliver a lecture on taking medication properly?

Further Reading

1. Pearce CJ and Byfield PGH. Free thyroid hormone assays and thyroid function. *Ann Clin Biochem* **23** : 230–237, 1986.
2. Woodhead JS and Weeks I. Circulating thyrotropin as an index of thyroid function. *Ann Clin Biochem* **22** : 455–459, 1985.
3. Editorial. Sensitive thyrotropin measurements: utility and futility. *Lancet* **i** : 1176, 1989.

15a

Scurvy Today

Vitamins are not a component of modern, heroic, high-tech medicine; that era passed some sixty years ago. But the general public remain extremely interested in them, and doctors should be too. If vitamins are not in the forefront of present day advances, at least not in those countries which are fortunate enough to possess an organised and affordable food supply, still they remain a component of a staggering number of diseases; indeed, probably every condition has some relationship to a vitamin requirement, imbalance, antagonism, interaction, or excess — even a broken collar bone (_inter alia_, sufficient vitamin C is needed for healing) or a splinter in the thumb (various vitamins are involved in the immune response.)

Vitamin C, otherwise known as ascorbic acid in its non-oxidised form, is well understood by all to be a component of fresh fruits and vegetables, and that these are a necessity in the diet. It is difficult to devise a diet devoid of the vitamin, but this can be achieved with highly processed or grossly-overcooked foods. Historically, the type of processing most necessary was preservation (drying, salting) and it was by this means that scurvy was the scourge of soldiers, and of sailors too when they began to make long voyages. Most doctors have never seen a case of scurvy. But _has_ it disappeared?

Plumbing Purple Spots

A fifty-year-old man complained of painful swollen feet and a rash consisting of itchy, purple spots about his arms. A history elicited only that he was a heavy drinker, without a job for the previous three years, and living alone. Physical examination revealed the the ankles were oedematous and the discoloration was found to be present also on the legs and abdomen. There was an enlarged liver and this was attributed to the alcohol. The first diagnosis was leukocytoclastic vasculitis, an inflammatory disease of the veins caused by neutrophils adhering to the endothelial surface, resulting in increased permeability and extravasation of red blood cells. This condition should however be manifested by increases in complement and cryoglobulin, which could not be detected. A battery of chemical tests were quite normal, but there was occult blood in the stool. On a second visit to the clinic, with a more thorough examination, it was noticed that there was a pronounced gingivitis (gum disease), and a corkscrew-like deformation of some of the body hair. This led to a revised diagnosis of scurvy, which was confirmed by a low serum vitamin C concentration of 5 μmol/l (normal range, 10–100 μmol/l).

In retrospect, the fact that the patient lived alone and was alcoholic could have alerted the physicians to the probability of a diet inadequate in fresh fruit and vegetables, and the ecchymoses (the purple discolorations), the gum infection and the hair deformation are all typical of scurvy. The basic lesion, probably, is degeneration of connective tissue within the vessel walls (probably a collagen defect) leading to the bleeding into the tissues, and into the gastrointestinal tract, as seen in this case. The extravasation of fluid is also evidently responsible for the oedema.

As has been mooted, in scurvy the hair follicles are also abnormal, being plugged with horny material (hyperkeratosis) and so there are subsequent hair deformities. The gum infection, which often confers a very bad breath, is probably due to bleeding round the gingival capillaries, for the same reasons as above.

In many cases, in the face of possible ascorbic acid deficiency, the doctors would not even bother to measure the vitamin in the blood, but quickly give a large oral dose, which will have a salutory effect on the various signs and symptoms in a few days if their suspicions are correct. Levine (Ref. 1 below) comments that it is still important to recognise scurvy (which can be a matter of some difficulty, as seen above, because it tends to mimic other diseases) if only because untreated patients may die. This in itself may be due to bleeding into the heart muscle.

ROLES OF ASCORBIC ACID

The exact molecular basis of the action of ascorbic acid is still somewhat unclear. However, there are probably multiple roles, such as:

(1) It participates in hydroxylation reactions by way of increasing activity of many hydroxylases (involved in collagen maturation, bile acid, carnitine and noradrenaline synthesis). Ascorbate does not seem to react with the enzyme protein like a true coenzyme; it may well keep metal cofactors for the enzymes in the reduced form, obligatory for their catalytic activity.

(2) It is a free radical scavenger, if only at relatively high concentration. Free radicals are compounds with one or more unpaired electrons and are thus highly reactive, avidly attacking compounds like membrane-bound unsaturated fatty acids, thereby abstracting electrons, and producing lipid peroxides, which are in turn unstable and decompose; free radicals can also damage nucleic acids.

Free radicals are produced by a large number of intracellular reactions. For example, neutrophils export the hydroxyl free radical into the space surrounding them, as a lytic agent for bacteria; it is important that this process does not go too far and damage the host tissues as well as the invader.

Electrons leak off the respiratory chain on to oxygen in mitochondria to yield the superoxide free radical, usually represented as $O_2^{\cdot}$
Ascorbic probably reacts with these free radicals before their damaging effect can go too far. Probably also it regenerates the reduced, scavenging form of vitamin E after it has been oxidised by free radicals.

(3) It has a role in immune function. The migratory response of neutrophils and macrophages appears to be enhanced by ascorbate. It also protects bystander lymphocytes against the bacteriolytic HOCl (hypochlorite, or bleach) generated by neutrophils (although this arm of its role in immune defence is more related to item 2 above).

MEGAVITAMINS

As we write Linus Pauling is still alive, now over ninety, taking several grams of ascorbic acid in a normal day and about 40 g when he feels a cold coming on, and still strenuously advocating the same for the rest of us. What he practises is so-called megavitamin dosage, defined as the ingestion of vitamins in synthetic or pharmaceutical form, in amounts which could not readily be gained from normal foodstuffs. For example, one of the richest palatable sources of vitamin C is the orange. If you wanted to ingest 1 g of the vitamin from this natural source you would have to eat about two kilos of oranges. This is not impossible, and far from impossible if the source of the 1 g is, rather, two or three kilos of a mixture of vitamin C-rich foodstuffs, such as citrus fruits, broccoli, black currants, cauliflower and cabbage. But if you decide, as many people do, that more is better, the impossibility of obtaining 3, 4 or 5g from natural resources becomes clear. (There is one fruit, the gooseberry-like Australian aboriginal bush-food *Terminalia ferdinandiana* which has a staggering 3 g ascorbic acid per 100 g. You would not need to eat much of this to obtain 3 g or even 10 g, but it is not available in the supermarkets.)

It is Pauling's contention that by not being able to synthesise vitamin C (like guinea pigs and other primates) we are suffering from an inherited disease of metabolism, having lost the enzyme gulonolactone hydrolase in our evolutionary history, presumably at a time when fresh vegatables and fruit were so plentiful a constituent of the diet that there was some survival advantage in avoiding an endogenous supply on top of the exogenous one. Thus because modern diets and cooking procedures cause a less than optimum intake of vitamin C, it is prudent to take supplements to bolster the immune system — to ward off the common cold, for example. The most controversial and serious aspect of the C megadose controversy applies not to the common cold, however — a side-issue which has all but disappeared from the medical literature in recent years — but to cancer. This was initiated by Pauling and Cameron who gave 10 g vitamin C daily to terminal cancer patients and observed an increased survival time as compared to matched controls.

The theory of its action refers to item 1 above. Since ascorbic acid is necessary for mature collagen synthesis via proline hydroxylation to hydroxyproline, it might thereby strengthen the fibrous capsule round a tumour and so limit its growth, or alternatively prevent the release of metastasising cells. Two subsequent studies in the Mayo Clinic did not substantiate the findings of Pauling and Cameron and an acrimonious debate ensued. Meanwhile, the epidemiological evidence on the subject has been steadily gathered. Workers in these studies had to work out some index of vitamin C content of diets and relate their calculations to statistics on cancers for the same populations. The evidence of a protective effect of the vitamin is said to be particularly strong for oral, oesophageal, gastric and pancreatic cancers. For hormone dependent cancers (ovary, endometrium, prostate and breast) there is little evidence of any benefit. Lung cancer is in a special category because most studies of its relationship to diet have concentrated on vitamin A (Chap. 15d); however, when the effect of C alone has been dissected out it has generally been thought to be protective. It is possible that vitamins C and A have a synergistic effect. Smokers, who are of course particularly prone to lung cancer, have definitely been established to be relatively vitamin C deficient due to a greater metabolic turnover of the substance.

So where do we stand? From many other points of view (the provision of fibre, vitamins A, B, E and K) everybody should be encouraged to eat fresh fruit and vegetables. But what of vitamin C in established cancer? It seems indefensible, as the clinical pharmacologist Louis Lassagna wrote, not to at least *try* substantial doses of vitamin C on cancer patients. Colorectal cancer, from which many of the patients in the direct intervention studies were suffering, is so resistant to chemotherapy that vitamin C, being cheap, plentiful and almost non-toxic, would be better than nothing. Also, failure with colorectal need not imply failure with all other cancers.

There is one other, more concrete aspect to the role of ascorbic acid in cancer, in that it blocks the formation of carcinogenic nitrosamines from nitrite. Nitrite itself is not used in foodstuffs but is formed from nitrates which are naturally present in some foodstuffs but also added to meat and fish as a preservative. Ascorbic acid reacts with the nitrite, especially at low pH and in the absence of oxygen.

VITAMIN C AND IRON

Seventy five percent of subjects with scurvy are anaemic, due to bleeding into the gastrointestinal tract, intravascular haemolysis and — unrelated to scurvy itself but to general malnutrition — a lack of iron folate and cobalamins in the diet. Under such circumstances, there will be a microcytic type of anaemia, but few megaloblasts. However, the lack of iron and ascorbic acid are related in that the vitamin is able to keep the metal in the reduced (ferrous) form, necessary for absorption in the gastrointestinal tract. That is the reason that oral iron medicines are always combined with vitamin C.

Further Reading

1. Levine M. New concepts in the biochemistry of ascorbic acid. *N Eng J Med* **314** : 892–900, 1986.
2. Block G. Vitamin C and cancer prevention. *Am J Clin Nutr* **53** : 270S–282S, 1991.

15b
Beriberi: An Old Asian Disease

SUDDEN UNEXPLAINED NOCTURNAL DEATH

Towards the end of the eighties, it became apparent that both migrant Vietnamese in USA and Thai construction workers in Singapore were prone to sudden unexplained nocturnal death (SUND). There were so many of the latter that in early 1990 the local press was asked to stop reporting them, to avoid completely destroying morale in the workers, who are badly needed to contribute to the island's booming economy. As the name implies, deaths always occur at night; room mates report that noisy breathing and gasping occur at the time of the crisis. Death can however be quite silent; one worker died quietly in his sleep on an overnight bus proceeding up the Malayan peninsula. Apart from intra-alveolar haemorrhage in some of the victims there were no abnormal findings at necropsy, and the only significant factor brought out by case control study was self-medication with traditional Thai herbal medicines. Additionally only men, not women, appear to be affected. It later turned out that similar deaths do habitually occur in the area of North East Thailand whence the workers come. The immediate cause of death has been termed ventricular fibrillation without underlying cardiovascular disease, that is, essentially an admission that it is unknown. The impotence of Western medicine was bidding fair to render the belief of the Thais themselves, that they are being visited by a malignant female spirit, just about as reasonable as anything else, were it not for an emergent idea that SUND represents a peculiar variety of beriberi.

As a result of thiamine, that is vitamin B1 deficiency, there are classically two types of beriberi — wet and the dry. It is not known why subjects develop one rather than the other. The wet type is a cardiomyopathy, the dry largely a peripheral neuropathy. The pathogenesis in either case is presumably related to the lack of B_1 for key enzyme reactions involving TPP, the coenzyme form of the vitamin (Fig. 39). In some ways the most important of the relevant enzymes is pyruvate dehydrogenase which provides two-carbon units to fuel the energy-producing citric acid cycle. In the absence of enzyme activity pyruvate accumulates and is partially reduced to lactate. The ensuing lactic acidosis appears to produce a vasodilation which increases cardiac output, but the heart itself suffers from energy deficit due to rundown of citric acid cycle substrate. A gross oedema can result. Nonetheless, there can be heart failure before the oedematous state is reached, in the form called shoshin beriberi (this being the Japanese for "damaged heart") formerly also prevalent in the Far East. If SUND is due to some sort of beriberi it is obviously the shoshin type, perhaps combined with genetic factors and stress.

A new chapter then may be about to be added to the history of beriberi investigation. Seventy to eighty years ago Hopkins, Funk, Eijkman and the other pioneeers of the vitamin theory found themselves with a severe credibility problem. Pasteur and Koch had heroically ushered in the age of microscopic pathogens and it came to be accepted that most diseases whose aetiology was unknown at that time would turn out to have a microbial basis. In the tropics, the vitamin theory must have seemed even more superfluous in the face of a host of parasitic diseases such as malaria, leprosy, diarrhoeas, filariasis, tuberculosis, and so on. It was natural that a further scourge — beriberi — might not readily be accepted as being due merely to a lack of minutely small quantities of something in the diet. But the struggles of Eijkman (who worked on beriberi in Java) were decisive. However, eighty years later, since gross vitamin deficiencies have all but disappeared in the areas round prestigious medical schools, it may well be that we are again in danger of neglecting the knowledge of nutrition so sorely won.

Unfortunately, if SUND is due to a type of beriberi, confirmation of it is not easy. As in most cases of vitamin assessment, mere analysis of the vitamin in the blood is thought to be unhelpful — better is a test of urinary excretion of thiamine in a four-hour period, before and after a test load of vitamin B1, especially if normalised against creatinine excretion. Of more interpretive value are carbohydrate loading tests, especially since lactate and pyruvate are easily estimated in modern laboratories, but the danger of a harmful surge of lactate might be a disadvantage, especially since shoshin beriberi has a definite association with lactic acidosis. Perhaps most applicable is the assay of the activity in red cells of transketolase (Fig. 39). This requires only a single sampling into a heparinised syringe, with the bonus of a complete aliquot of plasma for archiving, that is subsequent investigation of any component which may later turn out to be important.

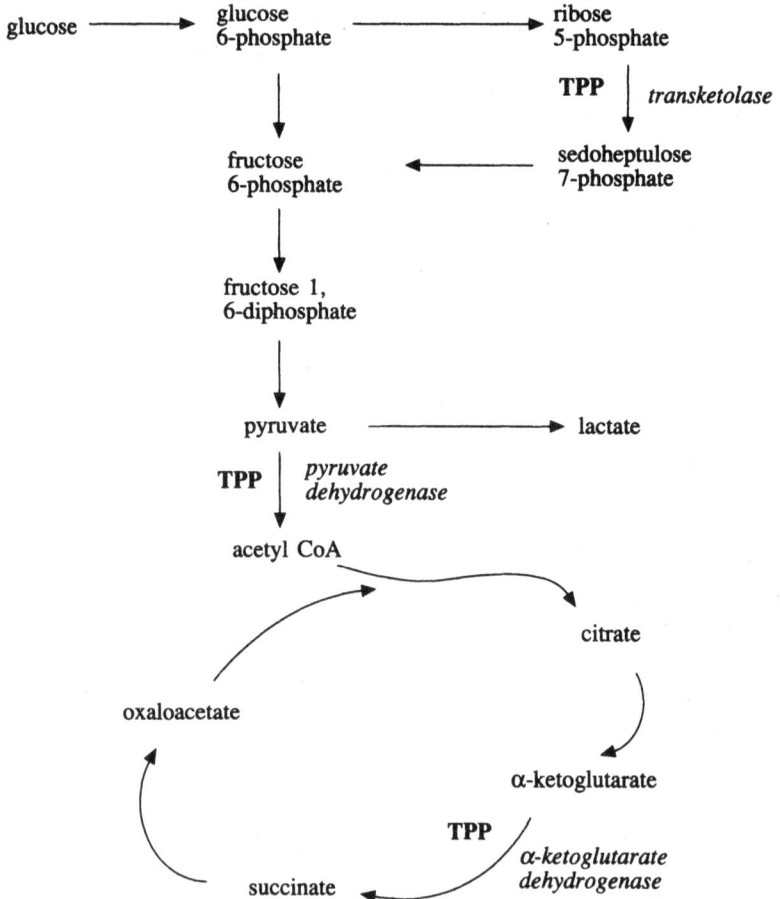

Fig. 39   Thiamine pyrophosphate (TPP) as a coenzyme in metabolism.

A single arrow may of course represent multiple steps, and the unidirectional arrows imply net utilisation of glucose as energy source.

TOTAL PARENTERAL NUTRITION (TPN)

Total parenteral nutrition, it is said, provides both opportunities and risks for patients. It might seem easy to concoct a nourishing soup to be pumped into the veins of the comatose patient, but achieving the exactly correct composition has proved to be a formidable task. Consider the following case:

An operation for a cancer in the gastrointestinal tract was perfomed on a sixty-year-old man, and necessitated subsequent TPN. Ten days later, he developed tachypnea, hypotension, and respiratory arrest needing intubation and mechanical ventilation. His arterial blood at that time showed the following picture:

pH	7.18		
pCO_2	16.2	mm Hg	(reference interval, 35–45)
HCO_3^-	5.4	mmol/l	(22–31)

Serum glucose at 8.4 mmol/l was only slightly elevated and the provisonal diagnosis of diabetic ketoacidosis was discounted. An estimation of lactate then gave 14.3 mmol/l (reference interval, 0.6–2.5). It was then suspected that the lactic acidosis might be due to an intraperitioneal abscess, but a second laparotomy showed no evidence of this. Despite mechanical ventilation and bicarbonate administration, his lactic acidosis continued to worsen and the TPN was discontinued. At this point it was realised that the pattern could be due to a deficiency of thiamine, which was immediately given as an intramuscular injection. Within five hours, his blood pH started to normalise and his cardiac status improved.

JUNK FOOD BERIBERI

Reports have recently appeared on a resurgence of beriberi in Japanese youths addicted to Western type fast foods, that is the hamburger/cola type diet. It may be that for genetic reasons the Japanese are more susceptible than others to thiamine deficiency, but be that as it may warnings have been put out about the need to question all patients closely about their diet if the signs of peripheral muscle weakness or impaired venous return are apparent.

ALCOHOLIC ATHIAMINOSIS

Alcoholics are prone to thiamine deficiency for several reasons.

(1) They tend to be malnourished per se.
(2) Absorption of vitamins from the gut is impaired.
(3) Conversion of vitamins to the coenzyme form in the liver is impaired.

A combination of these tends to produce psychoses of the Wernicke type (Chap. 18f) so that when all is said and done the signs and symptoms of thiamine deficiency are protean.

Summary

The vast majority of physicians practising today have never seen a case of beriberi, any more than scurvy. But from what has been written above, it is obviously useful to be able to recognise it when it occurs, possibly in:
   (1) Asian immigrants
   (2) Total parenteral nutrition
   (3) Junk food addicts
   (4) Alcoholics
Confirmation is possible by persuading the laboratory to measure transketolase in the erythrocytes, combined with any salutory effect of administering the vitamin itself.

Further Reading

1. Four letters in *Lancet*, dated May 12, 1990 (p. 1154), 12th May 1990 (p. 1154), June 16 1990 (p. 1471) and June 16 1990 (p. 1472)
2. Anon. Beriberi can complicate TPN. *Nutrition Reviews* **45** : 239–241, 1987.

15c
The Bs and Brains

"Taking supplements just gives you expensive urine."

— Victor Herbert
(quoted in Time Magazine, 6/4/92)

If your patient comes to you with capsules marked vitamin B_{15} and/or vitamin B_{17} and asks whether he should be taking more of them, you might be worried, because whatever may be the substances inside the capsules, they are definitely not genuine vitamins, and the latter at least is potentially highly toxic. It could be that your patient has picked up the capsules abroad, because they are banned by statutory authorities in many countries. Because of the complex nature of vitamin B nomenclature, and the fact that there are so many of them, a spurious one (or two) can be slipped into commercial preparations without most consumers being aware they are paying for something with no value whatsover. B_{15} (also called pangamic acid) and B_{17} (also called laetrile) were first marketed by a gentleman called Ernst Krebs (not to be confused with Hans Krebs of the citric acid cycle) who had isolated them from seeds and kernels; the first is a mixture of dimethyl glycine, a natural metabolite of choline, and gluconic acid; the second is a glycoside formerly known by the further name of amygdalin, isolated in the 19th century from almonds. It is this one which is particularly dangerous, for it contains cyanide which may be released from the parent glycoside by hydrolysis by mineral acid, such as hydrochloric acid in the stomach. This cyanide production was claimed as an anticancer treatment. There is no evidence for this, and several unfortunate people have died trying out the claim. Most respectable authorities would agree that there are 13 recognised vitamins (although some of them are constituted of groups of molecules of similar structure and activity):

A   (retinoids, carotenoids)
B_1 (thiamine)
B_2 (riboflavin)
B_3 (nicotinamide)
B_6 (pyridoxine)
B_{12} (cobalamin)
folate
pantothenate
biotin
C   (ascorbate)
D   (cholecalciferol)
E   (tocopherols)
K   (naphthoquinones)

The dilemma for the poor consumer (apart from the nomenclature, which is historical) is that each vitamin can be considered as holding infinite promise in one way or another, depending on who he listens to or what books and magazine articles he reads. He may be aware — confining consideration to the B-group for the moment — that classical medicine recognises thiamine therapy for beriberi; riboflavin for cheilosis and glossitis; nicotinic acid for pellagra; pyridoxine for neonatal seizures; folic acid and cobalamins (B_{12}) for megaloblastic anaemia, but that there are other, candidate areas, about which he would like concrete information.

CHILDREN AND B-VITAMINS

There is much concern that children, even in developed countries, may not be obtaining enough B-vitamins. Of course they are in no danger from frank beriberi or pellagra, but the idea that deficiencies may be subclinical, affecting performance at school, alertness, and capacity for physical exercise, or all of these and more besides, has been very persistent. It is compounded by fears as to excessive consumption of so-called junk foods. Beyond performance is reprehensible behaviour. The psychologist Schauss believes that aggressive behaviour in children is related to multiple mineral and vitamin deficiencies, athiaminosis being the most important among them. And of course, aggressive children are thought not to concentrate well at school.

In 1988, there was something of a furore when Benton and Roberts claimed that they had enhanced the non-verbal intelligence of a group of Welsh schoolchildren by giving them mutivitamin and mineral supplementation over an eight-month period. Another group from California hastening to do a comparable trial (there had been two entirely negative surveys in the meantime) gave their children either placebo or graded amounts of the nutritional supplement and subjected them to a wide battery of tests. Among these, non-verbal intelligence showed an improvement in the group supplemented by double the recommended daily allowance of the nutrients. Those given the largest amounts of supplement showed no difference from the controls.

Whatever the eventual outcome of such trials, and they could drag on for years if not decades, the upshot is that you will frequently be asked by parents whether or not they should give supplements to children who appear not to be doing too well at school. It is difficult to know what to say. If the parents are not well off, it is difficult to recommend that they buy supplements, knowing that the children, if they appear to be in good health, will merely excrete the vast majority of whatever is in the capsules. If there are sufficient means available to the family, who knows?

One golden rule is to check the preparations for their content of vitamins A and D, the ones most frankly toxic in excess.

B-VITAMINS AND NEUROPATHIES

Former prisoners of war who have been studied into old age still seem to show signs of the neuropathies resulting from (it is presumed) B-vitamin deficits in the camps. Of course thiamine deficiency shows a very characteristic neuropathy (dry beriberi, Chap. 15b) but the others — pyridoxine, nicotinamide, pantothenic acid, B_{12}, and folate equally have a supportive effect on the nervous system. Generalised deficiencies, associated with malnutrition, chronic infection, or pernicious vomiting, are characterised by symmetrical impairment of sensory and motor function, reduced reflex activity (usually more in the legs than in the arms) and often burning sensations, which may be quite painful. The progress of such neuropathies is undoubtedly slow, over months or years, but once detected, cure is almost immediate by means of parenteral or oral administration of a suitable cocktail of the Bs.

What of the more obscure neuropathies? There was formerly a disease called neurasthenia, or nervous exhaustion, characterised by a long list of signs and symptoms like headaches, irritability, poor memory, and vague aches and pains; Freud thought it was a manifestation of (usually) sexual frustration, as he would of course. There was an interesting sub-variety called tropical neurasthenia, very probably compounded of alcoholism, malaria and loneliness in those colonial officials posted up crocodile-infested rivers. The modern equivalents would be called neuropathies, neuralgias and dementias of unknown origin; massive amounts of B-vitamins have certainly been tried for them. It is not entirely "blunderbuss" therapy, being based upon the idea that in various diseases there may be enzymes or receptors defective in binding B-derived cofactors. If massive amounts of cofactor are synthesised through the agency of administered vitamin, the binding might be sufficient to support catalysis and correct the long chain of causation between molecular defect and clinical signs and symptoms. It has to be said, however, that megavitamin therapy finds no favour with the majority of reputable neurologists.

VITAMIN B$_6$ AND PREMENSTRUAL TENSION

It has often been commented with wonder in these pages that pathologies which must have been part of the human condition for millenia crop up in the fifties, sixties and seventies as "new" syndromes or diseases (the former term being applied to a group of signs and symptoms when the cause(s) remain obscure, multiple, or theoretical. The premenstrual syndrome was only fully described in 1953, by Greene and Dalton. Their success is testified by its use as a defence in murder trials. (In one such, the defence of premenstrual syndrome was disallowed by the judge in the crown court but accepted the Court of Appeal.)

Pyridoxine phosphate or vitamin B$_6$ was first tried out as a cure for the syndrome in the early seventies, on the basis that it is known to be a cofactor for the synthesis of the neurotransmitter serotonin, which seems to combat depression in some way. In any case, trials were mounted and have shown that among various populations of sufferers, there is usually a proportion of responders to B$_6$. The search will go on for a biochemical test to predict who these responders might be. For example, the serotonin metabolites in the urine might shown to be enhanced by a B$_6$ challenge.

NEURAL TUBE DEFECTS

Neural tube defects, encompassing spina bifida and anencephaly, are among the most distressing of congenital conditions and the idea that they could at least partially be prevented by vitamin supplementation in pregnancy was eagerly discussed when it was first mooted by Smithells. A number of trials took place to try to confirm or reject it. These were all retrospective — that is, samples of mothers who had, or had not, babies with neural tube defects were interviewed as to their vitamin intake during the pregnancy. Various statistical manoeuvres were performed to eliminate such variables as employment status, maternal education, income, race, prenatal care, and any other information which could be gleaned from the mothers. Of the three or four such surveys completed, a majority have indeed demonstrated a protective effect of "multivitamins". Since B vitamins are known to have a profound effect on neural tissues (above), there is the presumption that it is they rather than A, C, etc. which have the beneficial effect on the spinal cord. Certainly, until a prospective, controlled, randomised study is done, it seems only reasonable to give vitamin supplements assiduously to pregnant mothers. Again one has to be careful of vitamin A, which is teratogenic in some forms.

Comment

It was one of the triumphs of biochemistry to show how the minute amounts of the "accessory food factors" as they were called at the time, functioned as coenzymes. They are needed in such small quantities in the diet precisely because they have a catalytic function, e.g. for example nicotinamide adenine dinucleotide (NAD^+) from vitamin B_3 or nicotinic acid, is recycled millions of times during dehydrogenation reactions. An ingested molecule of glucose is used only once, for energy. But we still cannot relate the coenzyme-linked reactions to the integrity of brain and nerve cells.

Further Reading

1. Anon. Brains and vitamins. *Lancet* **337** : 587–588, 1991.
2. Anon. Evidence for an association between periconceptional use of vitamins and neural tube defects. *Nutr Rev* **48** : 23–25, 1990.
3. Brush MG and Hansen K. Pyridoxine in the treatment of premenstrual syndrome. *Br J Clin Pract* **42** : 448–452, 1988.

15d

Aspects of A

"The possibility of discovering anticancer substances which can be prescribed rather than carcinogens that must be proscribed is attractive ..."
— Sir Richard Doll

Vitamin A is a blanket term for a series of substances with common biological activity. It includes the carotenoids, the plant pigments which are split in the liver to the animal forms of the vitamin, which are therefore better described collectively as "provitamins A". Vitamins A per se are a group of retinoids, prominent among which are retinol (the alcohol), retinal (the aldehyde), and retinoic acid. An idea of the structure is essential for understanding their separate roles and synthetic analogues and is given in Fig. 40. Thus it appears that omnivores like most of us receive forms of the vitamin from both plant and animal sources. By far the richest source of the latter is liver, not by any means a daily component of the normal diet. Dairy products have considerable amounts, and probably most people in the West obtain the majority of vitamin A from milk, butter and cheese. The majority of the world's population, the Chinese, do not have dairy products in their diet; presumably their fondness for lightly cooked green vegetables in most dishes can supply sufficient amounts of vitamin A in the form of carotenoids.

Vitamin A deficiency runs a complex course, but the principal manifestions can be listed, in rough order of appearance, as:

(1) Nyctalopia (failure of dark adaptation).
(2) Follicular hyperkeratosis (horny plugs round the hair follicles).
(3) Bitot's spots (flakey lesions on the sclera).
(4) Xerophthalmia (corneal dryness and opacity).
(5) Immunodeficiency.
(6) Failure of reproduction (demonstrated only in animals but assumed to be transposable to humans).

The World Health Organisation has a complicated staging system to allow epidemiological assessment in areas where avitaminosis A is prevalent, like Indonesia.

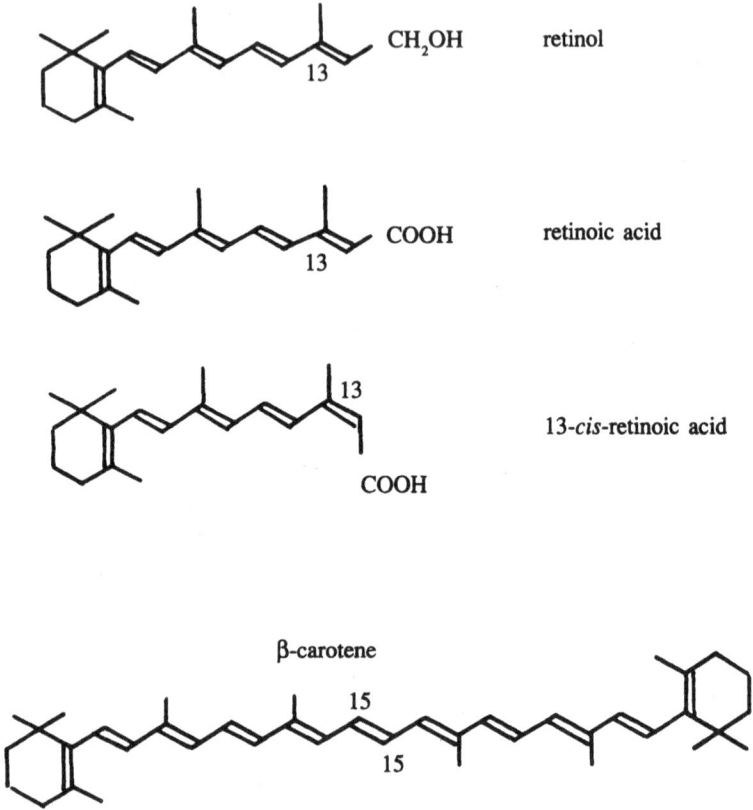

Fig. 40   Important forms of Vitamin A.

VITAMIN A AND BLINDNESS

The attack on the eye is one of the most distressing results of vitamin A deficiency, especially in children, and as noted above, it is a twin attack on the retina and sclera; this is in a sense fortuitous, for the two parts of the eye employ vitamin A for quite different purposes, the first as a component of a pigment in the visual cycle, the second in some way to maintain epithelial differentiation. The latter is much more fundamental, for after all, many animals get by very well without sight; some, such as bats and deep sea creatures have given it up as unnecessary. However, no species survives without orderly differentiation of squamous epithelia. Because the lesions of vitamin A deficiency usually occur in conjunction with marasmus or kwashiorkor, some like to refer to "blinding malnutrition."

VITAMIN A AND CANCER

Because:
(a) retinoids in some way make possible the differentiation of epithelial tissue
(b) cancer cells represent a loss of differentiation
(c) most cancers are epithelial cancers (carcinomas)
There is a prima facie case for investigating retinoid and carotenoid deficiency in cancer.

The first retrospective survey took place in 1975 and seemed to indicate a decreased rate of lung cancer in men with higher intakes of vitamin A. A more definitive study involved freezing serum from 16 000 men, identifying those who later suffered from cancer, identifying suitable matched controls for these, and analysing for vitamin A in the sera of them all. Further studies were not always entirely supportive, but overall, there was the impression that consumption of foods high in vitamin A is protective against colorectal and lung cancers.

VITAMIN A AND THE SKIN

Acne, at least in its milder forms, is nearly a universal human experience, and obviously involves a breakdown, in some sense, of the integrity of an epithelial tissue. The ultimate cause is unknown, but the horny plugs which form round the pilosebaceous duct block sebum flow and allow infection and infammation.

Topical and oral preparations of vitamin A in the form of all-trans retinoic acid (usually called tretinoin) were tried for the therapy of acne at an early stage and were found to be effective but too toxic. The pharmaceutical companies set to work to find more suitable analogues and trials of one of them, 13-*cis*-retinoic acid (isotretinoin) taken orally were successful. It is reported not only to suppress the acne, but also to prevent recurrence, even when the course of treatment has been terminated! It appears to reduce the rate of sebum secretion and keratinisation of the pilosebaceous duct. The snag is that patients taking it might either be, or become, pregnant, because of its marked teratogenicity.

The true excitement, however, was yet to come. Kligeman thought to try topical tretinoin not on acned, but on aged, sun-damaged skin. It appeared to stimulate new collagen and elastin synthesis, vascularisation, and epidermal renewal. It is one of the new hopes for ageing populations, like recombinant growth hormone (Chap. 14a).

It would be nice to know the biochemical basis of the efficacy of retinoids. Retinal or retinol are necessary for vision and reproduction, but they appear to be oxidised to retinoic acid for the maintenance of epithelia. In the sense that life itself can proceed in the absence of sight and reproduction, but maintenance of epithelia is of absolute importance for survival, then retinoic acid must have the most fundamental function.

VITAMIN A AND INFECTION

Early experiments involving vitamin A deprivation of animals revealed that sepsis generally followed blindness and growth retardation. The effect of the vitamin in preventing infection was ignored for many decades, however. In Java, Sommer established that there was a reduction in childhood mortality of about 34% in children who were given vitamin A supplements at a level of about forty times the recommended daily allowance in the West. This was attributable to protection against respiratory and diarrhoeal diseases.

Measles is thought to be particularly linked to vitamin A deficiency, as a viral disease which damages epithelial tissues throughout the body. In one trial in Africa, supplementation significantly decreased mortality from measles, especially in the under-two age group, and was especially protective in those children who developed laryngotracheobronchitis as a complication. It is not yet established, however, whether children living in areas with apparent sufficiency of dietary vitamin A should be given supplements as an immune support stimulant during infections.

TOO MUCH OF A GOOD THING

A man in his late twenties presented to his general practitioner with lack of appetite, weakness and lassitude. Subsidiary complaints were soreness round the mouth and anus, and some loss of scalp hair. Inspection confirmed this to be the case; further examination revealed that vital signs were all normal. Questioning revealed that he ate poorly, but he was vague about the exact nature of his diet. It seemed however that he liked to eat uncooked vegetables like carrots, broccoli and spinach. Haematological tests showed a mild hypochromic anaemia but the biochemical profile was normal except for a slightly raised aspartate transaminase.

The provisional diagnosis was malnutrition, possibly with multiple vitamin deficiencies. The patient was advised on dietary improvement, and offered psychiatric help, which was refused. He then disappeared from follow-up, but visited the same clinic after six months. By that time he had lost more weight, and the biochemistry results were more abnormal:

Aspartate transaminase	350 U/l	(reference interval, 0–40)
Gammaglutamyltransferase	510 U/l	(5–80)
Alkaline phosphatase	135 U/l	(40–120)

There was a pronounced hepatomegaly, and tests were conducted for hepatitis B antigen, which were however negative. A liver biopsy however showed a non-inflammatory cirrhosis. Since the patient claimed to be a non-drinker, it was thought that a possible cause of the cirrhosis might be vitamin A overdose, and on close questioning he admitted seeing a homeopath who prescribed 25 000 retinol equivalents (the modern unit) of vitamin A per day, advice which he had followed religiously for many months. The recommended daily allowance is about 1000 retinol equivalents. The plasma vitamin A concentration measured by high pressure liquid chromatography turned out to be about fifteen times the upper limit of normal. The subject was put on a low vitamin A (cereal) diet and his health gradually recovered.

The first cases of hypervitaminosis A were associated with overenthusiastic dosing of children with cod-liver oil. The symptoms are generally given as nausea, vomiting and headache. Bone overgrowth and liver cirrhosis are pathological findings. Both of these effects are probably due to transformation of cells to fibrolasts/osteoblasts by the action of the vitamin.

Vitamin preparations taken by patients should be checked to ensure that they do not contain vitamin A, at least in any large quantity.

Ingestion of massive amounts of the plant forms of the vitamin — giving hypercarotenaemia — appears to be benign. It is usually a result of the consumption of massive amounts of green vegetables or red palm oil; also, carrot juice is a common culprit with some food faddists. Hypercarotenaemia can be distinguished from jaundice by inspection of the sclera, which will look unpigmented; in jaundice of course the orange tinge is obvious.

Further Reading

1. Peto R, Doll R, Buckley JD and Sporn MB. Can dietary beta-carotene materially reduce human cancer rates? *Nature* **290** : 210–208, 1987.
2. Boyd AS. An overview of the retinoids. *Am J Med* **86** : 568–573, 1989.
3. Anon. Blind injustice. *Lancet* 1989.

15e

E for Ever

In the twenties when Evans and Bishop named a "hitherto unrecognised dietary factor essential for reproduction" it was quickly also dubbed the "antisterility vitamin", a misnomer when applied to humans but which the general public has consistently chosen to regard as a nomer. We now know it as vitamin E, or α-tocopherol in its principal chemical form, this last name deriving from one of the Greek words for birth. It is present mainly in vegetable foodstuffs, and after years of uncertainty its roles have been established as:

(1) *A free radical scavenger.* Vitamin E is a highly lipid soluble substance so it associates with biological membranes and interrupts the destructive action of free radicals, the highly reactive entities with one or more unpaired electrons (Chap. 15a). This intervention destroys the tocopherol molecule but it is probable that it can be regenerated by vitamin C. The membrane of the red blood cell is of course prone to free radical damage and a deficiency of vitamin E is manifested as haemolysis. A specialised aspect of its action is protection against free radical-generating drugs. Adriamycin, for example, is effective in cancer chemotherapy but its use is limited by severe side effects such as cardiomyopathy, which is a consequence of the free radicals it generates in the heart muscle. Such injury is aggravated by vitamin E deficiency.

(2) *Immune function.* It has been shown that human lymphocytes exposed to free radical generating systems suffered lower amounts of membrane lipid damage when vitamin E was present in the culture medium. This is related to the item above, of course, but renders in no doubt the importance of the vitamin in the immune response. More directly, the vitamin stimulates phagocytosis.

(3) *Neural function.* In monkeys, experimental vitamin E deficiency leads to loss of axons and/or myelin sheath in sensory nerves. The axons appear to accumulate lipofuschin — this is a pigment in nervous tissue derived from peroxidised fatty acids.

(4) *Reproductive function.* In male rats, mice, guinea pigs, dogs and monkeys, vitamin E deficiency results in immotility of the spermatoza, then degeneration of the germinal epithelium. In females of these species, there is

spontaneous abortion. No corresponding effects have been found in humans.

(5) *Muscle function.* Deficiencies of vitamin E in many animals is manifested as a myopathy, with an associated rise in serum creatine kinase. There is no unequivocal demonstration of the same pathology in humans.

Of course items 1–5 above may not be independent of each other. Free radical scavenging by vitamin E bound to membranes could protect nerve, gonads and muscle, besides many other tissues. Despite the numerous caveats with respect to humans, there is no doubt that vitamin E may be related to large number of diseases, despite the lack of a named deficiency syndrome.

HAEMOLYTIC ANAEMIA

This is the first, and very often the only, manifestation of vitamin E deficiency in humans. Where there is some other haemolytic problem, as in sickle cell anaemia, it would seem only prudent to ensure that the vitamin E status is adequate.

Haemolytic anaemia due to vitamin E deficiency in itself is however a real problem in premature babies (below).

MALAISE

Malaise is the opposite of well-being, the freedom from anxiety and fatigue, and the ability to enjoy social, artistic, physical and sexual activity. Vitamin E has been claimed to promote the quality of life, particularly with respect to the last two of this quartette, and the general public certainly buys capsules of it from health food shops to those ends. Are they to be advised to continue to do so? In one study, America college students were given vitamin E or placebo in a double blind study and asked to report on their sexual behaviour during the subsequent four weeks. There was no difference in activity between subjects and controls. Proponents of megavitamin therapy always claim, of course, that the dose was insufficient or the period of study too short. (A more cogent objection might be that it would have been better to do the trial on a group more in need of stimulation — college students are anyway so hyped up with respect to the matter in hand that a mere nutritional stimulus could hardly effect an increment, indeed it might be questioned whether an increment is possible at all). There have been rather more studies of the possible effects of vitamin E on athletic performance. It has to be said that none of these, if conducted according to acceptable scientific principles, has shown any improvement in speed or endurance. It has been commented often enough that the massive vitamin supplements given to athletes merely enrich the sludge in the sewerage works serving the training camps.

HEART DISEASE

An early study indicated that there were lower concentrations of the vitamin in the blood of those suffering from atherosclerotic diseases than in controls. There were then some intensive investigations as to whether it could affect serum cholesterol or triglyceride concentrations. There was no convincing demonstration of an effect on blood lipids in humans, although some contradictory results in rats and rabbits, and interest collapsed. It did not die however, and the whole topic was resurrected in a spectacular fashion by Oliver and others in 1991 after a study on men aged 35–54 in Scotland. They identified cases of angina pectoris, and matched them to suitable controls, upon which the blood of the whole group was analysed for vitamins A, C and E, as well as provitamin A, or carotenoids. It was shown that vitamin E was independently and inversely related to the risk of angina after statistical adjustment for a large number of confounding factors, such as smoking, weight, and so on. There was no evident protection from pro- or vitamin A, but a small one from vitamin C.

The theory of the efficacy of vitamin E in this context is as follows. When low density lipoprotein is peroxidised, it is taken up, not by the high affinity receptors which are found in almost all issues, but by macrophages, which become foam cells, contributing to the atheromatous lesion if they are situated in the artery wall. Vitamin E would interrupt this sequence at the very beginning, by removing peroxides and free radicals liable to react with the lipoprotein.

NEONATAL AND PAEDIATRIC PROBLEMS

In the 1950s, advances in neonatal care enabled very small premature babies to survive; they were fed formulas rich in polyunsaturated fatty acids and iron, which tended to generate a free radical load. (Fatty acid free radicals are derived from electrons donated by the iron.) Under such circumstances, when the body stores of vitamin E have not yet been built up by way of transfer across the placenta, a haemolytic disease can become apparent. It appears that breast-fed infants can achieve adult values of vitamin E more readily than those fed iron-rich artificial formulas .

Retrolentar fibroplasia, a blindness caused by an unruly mass of blood vessels over the retina, came to be associated with the oxygen therapy of premature infants because, in effect, oxygen free radicals are toxic to the developing eye. This simple explanation has been disputed for all cases of retrolentar fibroplasia but pre-emptive doses of vitamin E are still advised when there is likely to be hyperoxaemia.

In older children, there is often a neurological deficit rather than a haemolytic disease as a consequence of vitamin E deficiency. Once again, because medical advances enabled children with certain syndromes — in this scenario, various aspects of malabsorption — to survive, other hazards became apparent. Thus in cystic fibrosis, abetalipoproteinaemia, chronic pancreatitis, and biliary atresia, which are all associated with lipid malabsorption, vitamin E is not absorbed in the normal way, with the chylomicrons as a vehicle. The result appears to be either axonal damage or some failure of myelinisation such that there is hypotonia and absence of deep tendon reflexes and possibly a delayed ability to crawl or walk.

LIPOFUSCINOSIS

Detection of vitamin E deficiency in adults is very rare, but can be suspected if during routine histology, deposits of the brown fatty material called lipofuscin or ceroid are observed. This is better known in experimental animals and is thought to be a result of peroxidation of lipids in the mitochondria by free radicals, a process vitamin E prevents.

A 75-year-old man was admitted to hospital for a refashioning of a bile duct resection. Otherwise he was in good health considering his age. Previously he had chronic pancreatitis requiring total pancreatectomy and of course this requires re-arrangement of the plumbing in the area. A section of the duodenum taken for histology showed heavy deposits of ceroid in the smooth muscle (it fluoresces even in unstained sections). Since digestion was being maintained by enzyme administration, malabsorption was suspected, but no coherent history could be obtained by questioning the patient. Some estimations on his serum showed:

Albumin	37	g/l	(reference interval, 39–50)
Magnesium	0.74	mmol/l	(0.7–0.91)
Calcium	2.0	mmol/l	(2.1–2.6)

These indices of malabsorption are at the lower edge of normal so it seems most likely that it is fat or fat soluble vitamin absorption which is deficient. Some of the serum was sent to a specialist laboratory for vitamin E estimation; it was reported as 2.1 μmol/l, reference interval 11–35. The dosage of the pancreatic enzymes was adjusted, he was given vitamin E supplements, and remained well.

Further Reading

1. Bendich A. Antioxidant micronutrients and immune responses. *Ann N Y Acad Sciences* **587** : 169–180, 1990.
2. Howard LJ. The neurologic syndrome of vitamin E deficiency: laboratory and electrophysiologic assessment. *Nutr Rev* **48** : 169–177, 1990.
3. Riemersma RA, Wood DA, MacIntyre CCA, Elton RA, Gey KF and Oliver MF. Risk of angina pectoris and plasma concentrations of vitamins A, C and E and carotene. *Lancet* **337** : 1–4, 1991.

16a

Migraine: A Biochemical Headache

Who, reading pages such as these, has not had a biochemical headache? But a more universal biochemical headache goes by the name of migraine. Nearly everbody has gone through an attack at one time or another, for it is one of these very common yet obscure conditions, not least because clinicians have great difficulty in defining it and differentiating it from other forms of headache. It can be described, with little precision, as a familial disorder characterised by recurrent attacks of headache widely variable in intensity, frequency and duration. Attacks are commonly uni-lateral and are usually associated with vomiting, anorexia and nausea. Sometimes they are associated also with neurological and mood distrubances.

To complicate matters further, it can attack in a variety of forms. In classical migraine, the victim experiences an initial "aura" phase which can take the form of visual disturbance, like flashing lights (fortification spectra) and loss of parts of the visual field (central scotoma) in addition to paraesthesiae, and disorders of percep-tion and speech. These preliminaries are followed by the headache, vomiting and nausea phase.

Constriction of cerebral vessels is thought to be an important factor in the initial aura phase, with about 20% reduction in blood flow, leading to a degree of cerebral ischaemia and thus malfunction, followed by compensatory vasodilation and the intense throbbing headache, perhaps as a direct result of the stretching of pain sensitive vessels branching from the external carotid artery.

About thirty years ago, it was reported that 5-hydroxyindole acetic acid, the main metabolite of 5-hydroxytryptamine (5HT) also known as serotonin, is found in large amounts in the urine subsequent to an attack. Further, it turned out that serotonin is lowered in circulating blood platelets, which in the normal way have substantial amounts of it, during the attack itself. It is stored in their dense granules and avidly taken up by them from many organs including the intestine. Later, it was shown that during an attack, there is a circulating platelet serotonin releasing factor present in the blood. Thus platelet degranulation and serotonin depletion appears to be a feature of migraine attacks.

THE VASCULAR OR HUMORAL MODEL

The hypothesis is that released serotonin initiates changes in extracranial and cerebral circulation. A number of 5-HT receptors have been described (here the alternative name for serotonin is used) with various distributions:

5-HT1 — peripheral and central nervous sytems, with inhibitory effects on neural transmission; contraction of blood vessels.

5-HT2 — similar distribution to 5-HT1 except that they are excitatory on neural tissue and are also found on platelets, in which they elicit aggregation.

5-HT3 — peripheral nervous system, with an excitatory role.

The conclusion is that serotonin liberated from platelets can evoke a migraine attack by constricting cerebral vessels, after which it is catabolised and relatively depleted, this in turn causing dilatation and headache.

There are well-known dietary precipitants of migraine, like cheeses; they contain tyramine, another vasoactive amine chemically related to serotonin. Cheeses however do vary in their content — Camembert has about 2 mg /g and Stilton only about 0.45 mg/g. Chocolate is often rich in phenylethylamine, which like tyramine is able to release stored 5-HT and has a pressor effect on the cerebral vasculature (Fig. 41).

THE NEURAL MODEL

This suggests that the basic mechanism of migraine is to be found in the brain — stress and other factors result in an activation discharge from the hypothalamus leading to changes in the neurotransmission of the raphe nuclei and locus ceruleus. This results in changes in pain perception and in the cortical microcirculation. Since adrenaline, which is known to cause platelet aggregation and degranulation, is released from the locus ceruleus, there is here an evident overlap with the vascular/humoral model.

Anecdotal evidence in support derives from the reports by migraine sufferers of sudden and severe head pains after drinking something very cold, or eating ice-cream. In addition, so-called ice-pick pains — sudden and agonising jabs of head pain are also commonly experienced by migraine sufferers. These have all been ascribed to the hyperexcitability of the trigeminal nerve pathways (cranial nerve 5) which can relay impulses to the raphe nuclei and locus ceruleus. It has been termed the trigeminovascular reflex and an important neurotransmitter involved is probably substance P. Like other neuropeptides such as cholecystokinin it is important in vasoactive responses and pain perception.

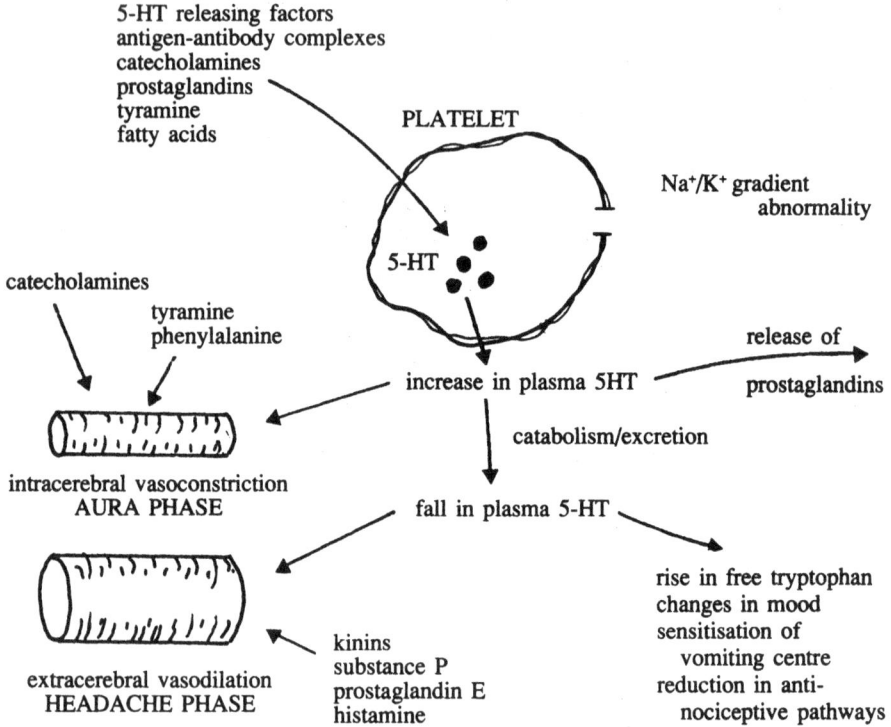

Fig. 41 Some factors in the pathogenesis of migraine.

THERAPEUTIC POSSIBILITIES

Methysergide, a 5-HT2 antagonist, has some potential in migraine, but unfortunately it has serious side-effects including retroperitoneal fibrosis. There are others available, including pizotifen, ketanserin and cyproheptadine. But some 5-HT1 antagonistic drugs have been developed, at present known only by serial numbers.

The 5-HT3 receptor seems to be less relevant, even though it has a role in the vomiting centre in the brain stem. The anti-emetic drug metoclopramide in high doses is capable of blocking 5-HT3 receptors. Glaxo have introduced another 5-HT3 blocker called Ondansetron which is also proving useful in the prevention of vomiting after cancer chemotherapy. This type of vomiting is a result of the cytotoxic agents releasing serotonin stored in the enterochromaffin cells of the intestinal tract. Serotonin stimulates 5-HT3 receptors in the vagus, setting up impulses relayed to the brain vomiting centre.

Further Reading

1. Crook M. Migraine: a biochemical headache?. *Biochemical Society Proceedings* **9** : 351–357, 1987.

16b
The Chemical Battle for the Mind

"Something has happened to me — I do not know what. All that was my former self has crumbled and fallen together and a creature has emerged of whom I know nothing. She is a stranger to me... she is not real... she is not I... she is I... and because I still have myself on my hands, even if I am a maniac, I must deal with me somehow.'

— Anonymous schizophrenia patient

It is said that at some time in their lives, about 1% of Western World adults are diagnosed as suffering from schizophrenia. That statistic translates into very large numbers of people. Biochemistry has little to offer in terms of diagnosis, which relies upon symptoms and signs resulting from the breakdown of the mental processes enabling us to distinguish our inner self from the world outside. Schizophrenia, *par excellence*, is a multifactorial disorder if not a group of loosely related diseases, so that looking for a single causative factor is not likely to be rewarding. Nevertheless, the neurotransmitter dopamine would seem to be implicated.

DOPAMINE CLUES

Post-mortem studies on brains from schizophrenia sufferers have shown abnormally high concentrations of dopamine in two areas of the limbic system, namely the anterior perforated substance and the nucleus accumbens with, in addition, an increased dopamine receptor concentration in the caudate nucleus. These would not seem to be post-mortem artefacts. Dopamine is mainly an inhibitory neurotransmitter, being found in slow conducting, small diameter neuronal fibres and thus disorders of dopamine in the brain may be expected to manifest neurological changes.

The use in schizophrenia of drugs such as chlorpromazine, described as neuroleptics (first used by French researchers to mean "that which seizes the neuron") has also indicated a major role for dopamine. Indeed, there is good correlation between the therapeutic efficacy of neuroleptics and their affinity to bind and blockade dopamine receptors in the brain, of which there are two types — D1 which is linked to cAMP signal transduction pathways, and D2 in which no such connection can be demonstrated.

Of the central catecholamine-containing neurones, dopaminergic neurones are amongst the most numerous, and tend to be arranged in a number of subtypes of particular topological projection, that is the nigrostriatal system which extends from the substantia nigra to the corpus striatum (globus pallidus, putamen and caudate nucleus) and is involved in the extrapyramidal motor control pathways.

The reason for this digression into the complexities of neuroanatomy is to help explain some of the extrapyramidal side-effects of neuroleptic drugs, such as their propensity to evoke Parkinsonian symptoms (Chap. 18b) which can be a limiting factor in their use in the treatment of schizophrenia. It is known that for optimal extrapyramidal function, the influence of the excitatory neurotransmitter acetylcholine and the inhibitory neurotransmitter dopamine need to be in balance. There is evidence that nigrostriatal dopaminergic neurones can inhibit cholinergic interneurones in the caudate nucleus and putamen. The cholinergic neurones in turn can excite gamma-aminobutyric acid neurones, which form part of a negative feedback loop to the substantia nigra in turn inhibiting dopaminergic neurones. In Parkinson's disease there is a significant decrease in the dopamine activity within the substantia nigra of the brain and consequent disinhibition of acetylcholine neurones. Thus by interfering with these pathways, neuroleptic drugs can elicit extrapyramidal side-effects, such as the limb rigidity and tremor characteristic of Parkinsonism. Interestingly, within another side-effect of neuroleptic drugs, namely tardive dyskinesia, the converse is seen, that is features of increased dopamine transmission and inhibition of acetylcholine pathways, within the extrapyramidal system. This probably results from chronic blockade of basal ganglia dopaminergic receptors leading to overactivity of dopaminergic synapses. It is likely that because of this long term blockade, there is an increase in expression of dopaminergic receptors and in an attempt to compensate. As a result, disturbances in the fine voluntary control of movement occur such as grimacing and the characteristic lip-smacking.

A further dimension of complexity in this aspect of neurobiochemistry is that the involvement of neuropeptide neurotransmitters has also been implicated. It used to be established dogma that only one neurotransmitter is released at each nerve ending. This has been disproved as in some instances, neuropeptide neurotransmitters are found together with conventional neurotransmitters within the same nerve terminal. Indeed, dopamine can be paired with cholecystokinin (suprisingly also found as a hormone in the intestine and capable of causing gall-bladder contraction) and acetylcholine with vasoactive intestinal polypeptide. It is intriguing that the brain and bowels have something in common! It has also been postulated that in the schizophrenic brain loss of cholecystokinin binding sites in the hippocampus region occurs. As cholecystokinin and related peptides are thought to inhibit limbic dopaminergic activity, it is conceivable that a disturbance in the cholecystokinin containing neurones could result in hyperactivity of dopaminergic systems.

Thus there is a complex system of neuronal connections and neurotransmitter pathways in the brain which can become unbalanced in disease (Fig. 42) . A few

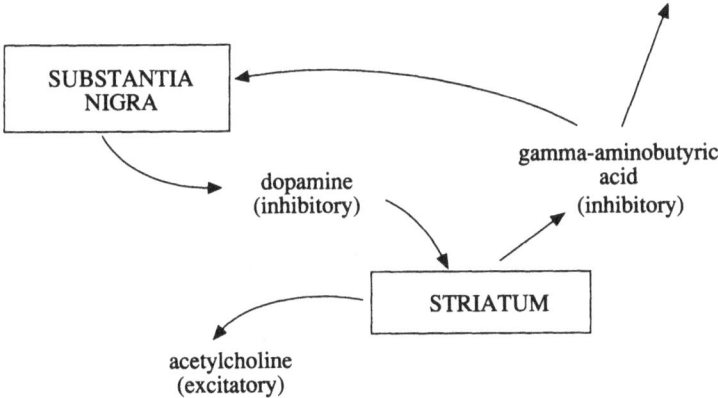

Fig. 42 The interaction of neurotransmitters in the extrapyrimidal tracts.

An interaction of at least three neurotransmitters is involved in motor control. The inhibitory dopaminergic neurones balance the excitatory cholinergic ones, but there is also an inhibition by gamma-aminobutyricergic neurones of the striatum on the substantia nigra and (ultimately) on the higher centres of the brain. In Parkinson's disease there is thought to be degeneration of the dopaminergic neurones of the substantia nigra leading to the characteristic tremors.

examples have been described in the case of schizophrenia. Hopefully such studies will aid the treatment of this disorder, although the observation of a possible genetic connection related to chromosome 5 needs also to be explored.

CLINICAL IMPLICATIONS

(1) Research is progressing into the further biochemical dissection of neurotransmitters in schizophrenia. This obviously has a bearing upon potential therapeutic agents.
(2) Family and twin studies being carried out on schizophrenia suggest a genetic component.
(3) The complex interplay between brain neurotransmitters has implications in other disease states involving the brain.
(4) Beware of the possibilities of extrapyramidal side-effects in patients on neuroleptic drugs, which can be explained by these interrelationships among the brain neurotransmitters.

Further Reading

1. Reynolds GP. Beyond the dopamine hypothesis. *Br J Psychiatry* **155** : 305–316, 1989.

16c
The Third Eye, the Seat of the Soul and Jet Lag

Descartes with his usual intuition about essentials designated the pineal gland as the seat of the soul, and no doubt would hardly be surprised at the resurgence of interest in it at the present day. For in humans at least, it had long been thought of as a vestigal organ, with no detectable functions. The situation is rather different in many other species — in lower vertebrates and some birds, the pineal gland is almost certainly important in regulating circadian neuronal circuits, while in some mammals it is involved in the processing of information concerning day length (also called photoperiod). This latter function, as a "third eye" is obviously important in species in which there is seasonally-controlled reproductive behaviour.

The response to day length is mediated by the neurohormone melatonin (N-acetyl-5-methoxytryptamine), secreted by the pineal gland. This is a substance derived from 5-hydroxytryptamine (5HT) or serotonin, and a look at the structures of these compounds suggests correctly that they are derived ultimately from the amino acid tryptophan. The rate limiting enzyme for the synthesis is serotonin N-acetyl transferase, whose activity is at least least fifty times greater during the night than in the day. The activity of the enzyme catalysing the O-methylation step also seems to be dependent on the time of day. The upshot is that even in humans, melatonin is mostly synthesised at night.

As usual, the details of the pathways regulating the entire synthesis are complex and incorporate many neural mechanisms. The increased activity of the rate-limiting enzymes at night is partly controlled by noradrenaline activity acting upon beta-adrenergic receptors, and released by post-ganglionic sympathetic neurones derived from the superior cervical ganglion. Suppression of synthesis by light is by way of a pathway from the retina to the retinohypothalamic tract and the suprachiasmatic nucleus, thence to the pineal. The suprachiasmatic nucleus plays a central role in the generation of circadian rhythms and has been frequently termed the "central clock", the fine adjustment of which is by the dark-light cycle.

SAD TO RELATE

Psychiatrists are interested in melatonin in the context of affective disorders, which in very broad terms encompass depression and mania. A typical person with the rather serious diagnosis of manic depressive psychosis has a bout of depression for a few weeks and spontaneously recovers. Then there is a relapse during which he is either excited, elated and talkative (a manic phase), or miserable, pessimistic and inactive. Depressive illness is distinguished from manic depressive psychosis on somewhat technical grounds but the typical patient becomes generally less interested in events, withdrawn, tired and irritable, with loss of appetite, weight and libido. *He feels worse in the morning and better towards evening. He can fall asleep on going to bed, but wakes in the early hours and cannot nod off again.* In mania, there is some sort of enhanced activity in a number of areas, with *reduced need for sleep.* Note the italicised sleep- and time-related factors. It is a moot point as to whether the depression and sleep disturbance common to students round about examination times constitute a mild form of these syndromes.

Another important observation that hints at an involvement of melatonin in some affective disorders is that some forms of depression show a seasonal distribution, with peaks of depression occurring in autumn and spring. It has been proposed, therefore, that this could be related to rapid changes in day length during these periods and that changes in the light-dark cycle may alter circadian rhythm patterns, particularly at the equinoxes.

Melatonin is thought, with more substance, to be a culprit in a variety of depression with a marked temporal component, that is seasonal affective disorder (SAD) sometimes also known as winter depression. It is recognised by psychiatrists in North America but does not yet appear in the International Classification of Diseases. It can be a complicated disorder with a bipolar component, described as episodes of depression in winter but some degree of mania in springtime. In any case, it has been proposed that there is a disruption in the rhythm of melatonin secretion rhythm in SAD sufferers as compared to normal individuals. Treatment programmes have been devised by manipulating the light exposure — one such regime attempted to create an artificial summer by exposing the patient to full-spectrum bright light in the evening and morning, in the hope that altering the melatonin rhythm pathways would improve symptoms. Although some measure of success was claimed, other more critical researchers suggested a placebo effect.

The evidence for a role of melatonin in the disorders just described would be fairly described as circumstantial were it not for the fact that some anti-depressant drugs such as monoamine oxidase inhibitors and brain amine uptake inhibitors, like desmethylimipramine do increase melatonin production by the pineal gland. Moreover, serotonin as a melatonin precursor is functionally deficient in some depressed patients. We may thus soon expect to see melatonin on the laboratory request form as one of the few biochemical tests with a direct relevance to psychiatry. It is possible however that the metabolite 6-sulphatoxymelatonin will be more useful. It can be measured in a twenty-four hour urine collection, which serves as a sink for the day's melatonin production and eliminates short term pulses in secretion as a distorting factor.

Therapeutically, melatonin could find a place in the treatment of certain depressive disorders, although at present this remains hypothetical and needs further research. However, exogenous melatonin has been used to reduce the mood changes experienced by some jet-lagged travellers flying across at least eight time zones. Presumably, their dark-light brain patterns and circadian rhythms become confused. (You will know that the research now going on has come to some fruition when the flight stewardess gives you a melatonin capsule along with your coffee.) More seriously, the substance has also been tested a resynchroniser of disrupted sleep in totally blind subjects, and as a pace-setter for patients suffering from delayed sleep phase syndrome, a condition in which they combine severe insomnia with an inability to fall asleep at a desirable clock time.

Further Reading

1. Arendt J. Melatonin: a new probe in psychiatric investigation. *Br J Psychiatry* **155** : 585–590, 1989.
2. Thompson C, Stinson D and Smith A. Seasonal affective disorder and season-dependent abnormalities of melatonin suppression by light. *Lancet* **i** : 703–709, 1990.

17a

The Interferons

"Although the names of peptide regulatory factors are often misleading, there are few problems provided everybody adopts the same misnomer for the same molecule ..."

— AR Green (from Ref. 3 below)

Antibiotics revolutionised the fight against infectious disease but proved to be almost valueless aginst viruses. The interferons were discovered in the 1960s as products of cells infected by viruses, and were shown to be inhibitory ("interferent") of virus replication, so great hopes were raised that they might fill in the huge therapeutic void thus created. The name "interferon" was felicitous — it is highly descriptive and easy to remember, and the potential of the discovery caught the imagination of medical journalists, who wrote of its promise for many years. The great hopes are only now, thirty years later, beginning to be realised, but not in respect of virus infections; concomitantly, it has been recognised that interferons are only one of a large class of substances called **cytokines**.

As the separate members of each cytokine series was discovered, their names were serialised; thus we have interferons α, β, and γ, and the interleukins 1, 2, 3, etc. The outcome of this method of nomenclature can be unfortunate — one is reminded of the B-vitamins, which were also serially named, as B_1, B_2, B_3, and so on. However at the present day although there is a B_{12} there is no B_7, for example. What was originally so named turned out to be a mixture of several of the others, and the anomalies have given trouble ever since. In the same way, haemopoietin-2 turned out to be the same as interleukin-3; and interferon-β-2 the same as interleukin-6. There is no doubt then that with increasing knowledge the nomenclature of the cytokines will further shift. They are about to become important as prescription drugs, so more easily remembered names will presumably be introduced by the pharmaceutical companies. (Interleukin-2 is on the verge of being marketed as Proleukin by Cetus, a bioengineering company, for example.) In the meantime, a sort of classification is as follows:

    (1) Interferons — the class of cytokines originally discovered to protect cells against viruses.

(2) Interleukins — primarily involved in the immune response.

(3) Colony stimulating factors — primarily related to haemopoiesis.

(4) Tumour necrosis factors — substances cytotoxic to animal tumours (also called cachectins because they are thought to be involved in the loss of appetite in cancer patients.)

(5) Miscellaneous cytokines — platelet-derived growth factor comes under this category.

It is not a tidy categorisation — how can it be in the face of the sort of crossover nomenclature mentioned above? Moreover, some of the cytokines share, not the same name, but some of the same functions; in other functions, they are disparate. Further, the effects of a specific cytokine on a single cell type are not immutable, but vary depending upon priming or sensitisation effects by other molecules. This appears to happen when a receptor alters the cellular distribution or binding affinity of a receptor for some other cytokine, so-called transmodulation or "receptor cross-talk".

The compounds under item 2 above are the subject of the next section (17b) and platelet-derived growth factor of the one after that (17c). Item 3 above is substantially dealt with in Chap. 13b since the main clinical application, at the moment, is in nephrology.

At least they all have something in common in that they are large polypeptides or proteins, whether glycated or non-glycated. In addition, they are all paracrine or autocrine in their activity, not endocrine — they act principally in the area immediately surrounding the cell which synthesises them, or even on the synthesising cell itself. On reflection it is obvious that cells must be able to signal to each other at close range — for example, epithelial cells in the skin grow in concert, respecting each other's space, refraining from crowding out neighbours. Once the concept is accepted, the application of mature knowledge can obviously be applied, inter alia, to :

(1) Enhancement and control of cell proliferation in wound healing.

(2) Promotion and control of haemopoiesis.

(3) Activation and control of the immune response.

("Control" is emphasised because all biological processes can go too far: too massive a cellular response in wound healing leads to keloids; in haemopoiesis to haemocytosis, and in the immune respose, to allergies and anaphylactic shock.

INTERFERONS TODAY

There are three main types, named α, (or leukocyte), β (fibroblast), and γ (so-called immune, from T-cells).

The first of these comprises 15 sub-members, the other two are unique in themselves. One of the modes of action is to induce (2',5')-oligoadenylate synthetase which polymerises ATP to give an oligonucleotide with the capacity to activate cellular RNAse. Viral RNA is thus broken down.

It was established at an early stage in the AIDS epidemic, however, that the interferons are not effective against the HIV virus. But the spectrum of activity of interferons goes far beyond virus inhibition anyway — they are anti-mitotic for many cancer cells, stimulators of natural killer cells, and apparently pyrogenic, i.e. fever-producing.

INTERFERONS AND THE CLINICIAN

Interferons can be made either by classical techniques of protein separation or by recombinant DNA methods. However as they are proteins they cannot be given by mouth, rather by the intramuscular, intravenous or intranasal routes. Intensive trials have highlighted the following applications of interferon-α:

(1) *Hepatitis.* Patients with chronic hepatitis B infection, which carries with it a predisposition to hepatoma, respond with lowered serum transaminase activity, as a marker of reduced hepatocellular damage. It remains to be ascertained whether the drug can rid the liver of the virus and if so, in what proportion of patients.

(2) *Hairy cell leukaemia.* This is characterised by splenomegaly and the presence, in the serum and bone marrow, of B-lymphocytes with peculiar "hairy" projections, and shows a response rate of almost 90% to interferon- Unfortunately this disease has a long natural course so the effect on long term survival is not yet known.

(3) *Chronic granulocytic leukaemia.* This slow proliferation of long-lived granulocytes and progressive bone marrow failure has also been successfully treated.

(4) *Multiple myeloma.* This, the uncontrolled proliferation of lymphocytes producing a monoclonal antibody does not respond to interferon-α but it may be possible to use it as an adjunct to other therapies.

(5) *Kaposi's sarcoma.* The by now well-known lesion of the skin and the gastrointestinal tract in AIDS responds to inerferon-α in about two fifths of cases.

Each of these applications has a limited success rate, and side effects have of course been extensively documented. Interferons-β and -γ have no advantages, so far, over α. None have been shown to be useful for solid tumours except for the occasional, dramatic cure in cases of malignant melanoma and renal cell carcinoma.

Further Reading

1. Windebank KP. The cytokines are coming. *Arch Dis Childhood* **65** : 1283–1285, 1990.
2. Galvani D, Griffiths SD and Cawley JC. Interferon for treatment : the dust settles. *Br Med J* **296** : 1554–1557, 1988.
3. Green AR. Peptide regulatory factors: multifunctional mediators of cellular growth and development. *Lancet* **i** : 705–709, 1989.

17b

Interleukins

Interleukins can be described, at least as a first attempt, as regulatory polypeptides produced by lymphocytes and macrophages. Some of them can originate from cells without immune function and other cytokines like tumour necrosis factors, interferons and colony stimulating factors (depending on their origin and activity) may also fit the description. At the present time, there are about nine interleukins. The biochemical input was to purify and sequence these factors once they were detected, then to identify and clone the genes for them. A challenge at the present day is to explore and understand the nature of the sugar attachments they bear, and the regulation of the high affinity cell surface receptors with which they interact. Sugars are not present on the products of the cloned genes, but they are still biologically active, so that the glycation process must have some quite subtle basis.

Interleukin-1 is a secretory product of the macrophage (and as is now known, other cells) which supports thymocyte (T-lymphocyte) proliferation in culture. Its biological effects are very diverse — indeed it has the broadest spectrum of all the interleukins. One publication (Ref. 1) lists no fewer than 34 of them, encompassing very diverse cells and tissues. As a generalisation, it can be said to promote antigen-specific immune responses, inflammation, and the remodelling of extracellular matrices. In respect of the last of these, it induces cells to release proteoglycanases, collagenases, and gelatinases which are involved in connective tissue lysis. Its role in disease must be profound, yet awaits clarification.

Interleukin-2 was first found as a substance causing massive proliferation of lymphocytes. It was later ascertained that the lymphocytes in question are killer T-cells, derived neither from the T- or B-cell lines, and having the power to lyse virus-infected cells, cells originating in the bone marrow, and tumour cells. It was the last of these which was seized upon as a potential therapy, and it was soon shown that the leucocytes of some cancer patients produced less interleukin-2 than controls. There were then early efforts to administer it in the hope that it would selectively attack cancer cells, but these were unsuccessful. However, when killer T-cells taken from patients with malignant melanoma were grown in vitro in the presence of interleukin-2 and then reinjected along with more interleukin-2, there was some success — one patient was dramatically cured, and in most of the others there was a degree of tumour regression.

Interleukin-3 is a colony-stimulating factor, that is it induces the proliferation of haemopoetic cells, and so has some similarities to erythropoietin (Chap. 13b).

Interleukin-6, distinguished by no less than ten separate names in 1986–87, until various groups of investigators realised they were intent on the same protein, is produced in large amounts not just by T-cells, but by endothelial cells and mast cells, as well as cervical and bladder cancer cells. It is a heterogeneous product by virtue of variations in O- and N-glycation of the polypeptide chain. Its expression is induced by virus infection and by other cytokines and it has the diversity of effects; these can however be rationalised as a response to injury. It stimulates ACTH secretion, for example, which in turn renders available the anti-stress adrenocorticoids. It is a colony stimulating factor. Moreover, it is the main effector for the acute phase response. This is a result of infection, injury or malignancy, and is characterised by fever, negative nitrogen balance, leucocytosis, vascular permeability, and enhanced synthesis of a number of glycoproteins in the liver. These last are the acute phase proteins.

ACUTE PHASE RESPONSE AND CYTOKINES

Interleukin-6 seems to be instrumental in modulating the acute phase response, with interleukin-1 and tumour necrosis factor playing subsidiary roles. This newer knowledge has extended the scope for clinical chemistry investigation, which previously centred on the serum concentrations of certain liver-derived proteins, primarily C-reactive protein, which is only detectable in significant amounts in injury and inflammation. (It was so named because it has the ability to co-precipitate with pneumococcal C-polysaccharide.) Subsequently other proteins were found to be raised in the serum in the acute phase (Fig. 43); some, such as albumin, transferrin and the apolipoproteins, on the other hand, are decreased and were called negative acute phase proteins.

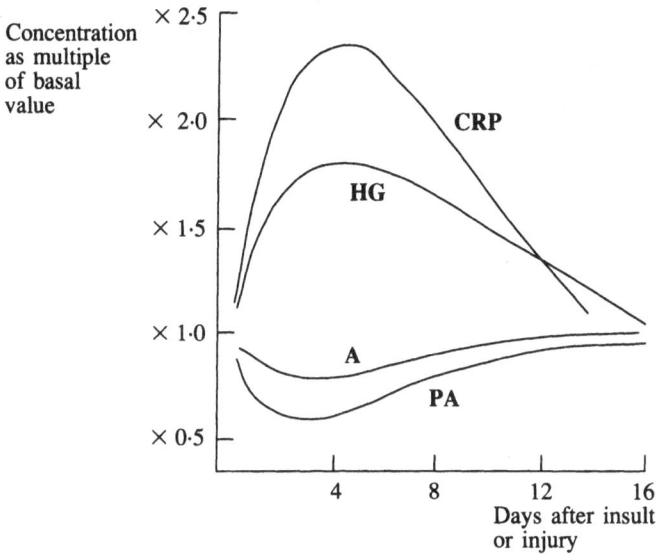

CRP = C-reactive protein; HG = haptoglobulin; A = albumin; PA = prealbumin.
The latter pair can be termed negative acute phase proteins.

Fig. 43 Some proteins of the acute phase reaction.

Measurement of the acute phase proteins is not used for diagnosis, rather to monitor the response to therapy (e.g. by antibiotics) and to try to detect complications, e.g. incipient rejection after a kidney transplant. We will see the assay of interleukins gradually replace that of the acute phase proteins in the course of attempts to follow (and then respond to) the course of inflammation in individual patients.

Comment

In trying to understand, let alone write about, cytokine biology one has a persistent sense of the inadequacies of the human mind. One can only hope that unifying concepts will arise as immunologists sort out the cytokine-mediated responses of different populations of cells and the type of novel estimations we should be offering to physicians will become apparent. Some of the presently known interactions are suggested in Fig. 44.

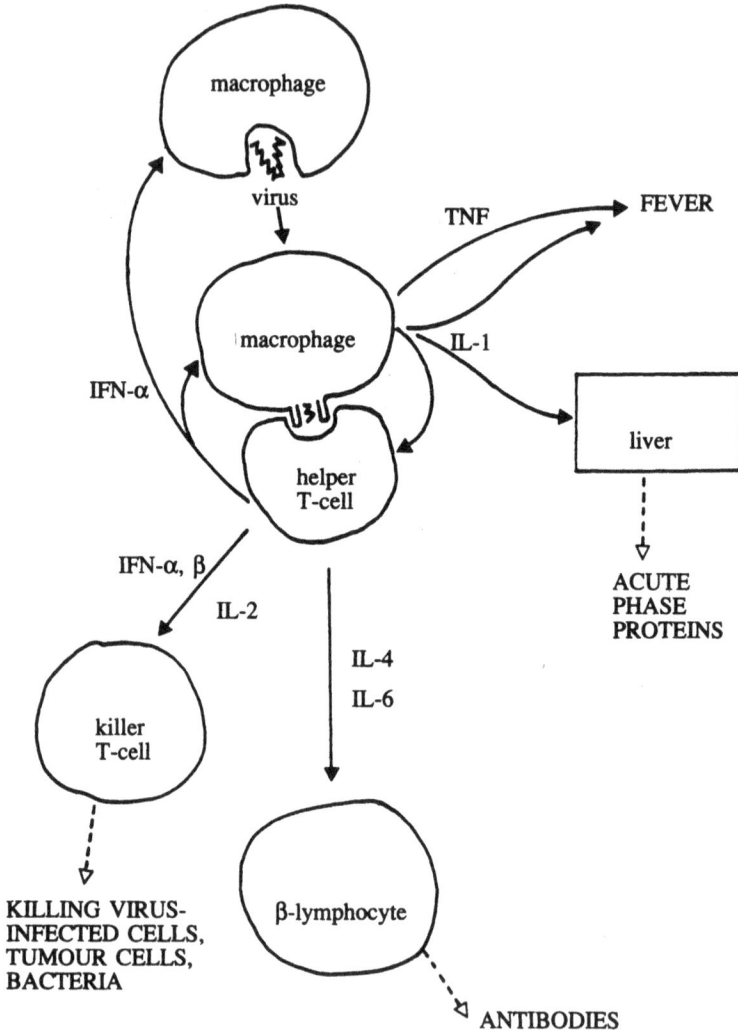

Fig. 44 Some actions of cytokines.

A macrophage ingests and digests the invader, exemplified here by a virus. A fragment of the invader becomes the "processed" antigen, expressed on the surface of the macrophage in conjunction with the major histocompatibility complex. This assemblage is recognised by a receptor on the helper T-lymphocyte. Such a train of events triggers off the synthesis and release of cytokines, whose effects will include fever, the acute phase reaction, the synthesis of antibodies, and the activation of killer T-cells.

Further Reading

1. Whicher JT and Evans SW. Cytokines in disease. *Clin Chem* **36** : 1269–1278, 1990.
2. Arai K, Lee F, Miyajima A, Miyatake M and Yokota T. Cytokines: coordinators of immune and inflammatory responses. *Annu Rev Biochem* **59** : 783–836, 1990.

17c
Platelet-derived Growth Factor

A REMINDER ON PLATELETS

The platelet or thrombocyte is a small elliptical fragment of the cytoplasm of the megakaryocyte. The main function of platelets was thought until recently to be the formation of the haemostatic plug after injury. They have the capacity to stick to surfaces, except the pristine endothelial surface, which is not recognised by them as a product of trauma or injury. If it is damaged, however, the situation is entirely different. But the discovery that platelets have functional receptors and secrete enzymes, growth factors, and coagulation proteins has caused a revision of this concept of an essentially passive role. The secretion of platelet-derived growth factor (PGDF) originally shown to support the growth of cultured cells when platelets were added to the medium, in itself gives them an effector function.

PLATELET-DERIVED GROWTH FACTOR (PDGF)

PDGF was originally isolated from platelets with much difficulty, for one platelet has only about 1200 molecules of the substance. Moreover, the cationic nature of PDGF renders it liable to stick to glass as well as damaged tissue surfaces, necessitating the use of potentially destructive solvents and detergents for its extraction. Within the platelet PDGF is located in the alpha or protein storage granules, although synthesis almost certainly originally occurs in the parent megakaryocyte, which explodes in the lungs to produce the platelets. However, other cells also express PDGF-like substances, including vascular smooth muscle cells, so the substance might well be important for myogenesis. In addition, there is evidence that macrophages/ monocytes and vascular endothelial cells also produce a compound at least similar to PDGF. Interestingly, some tumour cells, such as human osteosarcoma, also secrete growth factors with some similarity to PDGF.

Platelets however are undoubtedly an important source of the compound; it is released from them by agents like collagen, ADP and thrombin. These are prominent at sites of wounding and necrosis, and so the interaction is undoubtedly of relevance to repair mechanisms. This idea is supported by the fact that PDGF has a short plasma half-life of less than two minutes, implying a local effect round the site of the injury, as opposed to a systemic one. It is a protein of molecular weight of about 30 000, consisting of two polypeptide chains (A and B) connected by disulphide bonds. The dimer structure is essential for biological activity, with the A-chain having a molecular weight of about 18 000 and the B-chain of about 16 000. The carbohydrate linked by N-glycosylation to the A chain may account for the strongly cationic nature of PGDF.

A point that has raised considerable attention is the structural homology of the PDGF B-chain to that of the gene product of the oncogene *v-sis* of simian sarcoma virus. This is important as it hints at the oncogenic potential of some cytokines, in this case PDGF. Fibroblasts, say, when infected with the simian sarcoma virus become committed to producing unchecked amounts of a very active growth factor.

If PDGF is physiologically active, it should have a receptor, which indeed has been described on fibroblasts, glia cells and smooth muscle cells, although not on endothelial cells, the ones the platelet mostly comes into contact with. However, this is in accord with their activity only in damaged blood vessels and tissues. The PDGF receptor of fibroblasts is a 185 kilodalton glycoprotein spanning the plasma membrane of the cell. The receptor binds PDGF quite specifically, although it is similar to the receptor for macrophage colony stimulating factor and also to another oncogene product, namely *v-kit*.

INTRACELLULAR SIGNALLING AND PDGF

Probably the main event resulting from PDGF binding to its receptor, and which initiates the cellular response to PDGF, is tyrosine phosphorylation. The amino acid tyrosine, (see Chap. 9c) can undergo phosphorylation catalysed by tyrosine kinase, and is an important regulatory process in cells. The substrate for tyrosine kinase, upon activation by PDGF binding to its cell receptor, is a 42 000 molecular weight protein, which is rapidly phosphorylated, but how this phosphorylated protein evokes a mitogenic response remains to be elucidated.

The result of activation of the PDGF receptor is an excellent example of a biological system utilising a number of signal transduction processes. One of them is the breakdown of phosphatidylinositol biphosphate to form inositol triphosphate (IP3) and diacylglycerol. These are both active compounds in that IP3 can cause an increase in free intracellular calcium levels by mobilisation of calcium from intracellular stores. Calcium in turn can activate protein kinase C. Diacylglycerol is also thought to activate protein kinase C, which in its turn can modulate the activity of certain proteins. The cleavage of phosphatidylinositol biphosphate is catalysed by the rate-limiting enzyme phospholipase C, which is controlled by guanine nucleotide binding proteins, called G-proteins. There is a series of such proteins capable of regulating protein responses, usually either with activating or inhibitory roles. G-proteins are membrane-bound heterodimers, composed of an alpha subunit that binds the guanine nucleotide and a beta-gamma dimer. The alpha subunit also has intrinsic GTPase activity, thus it is able to breakdown GTP and thus terminate the reaction involving GTP binding. You will recognise all this as mainstream biochemistry. Unfortunately, at the present time the cause and effect chain peters out at some point between the cytoplasmic events described and the mitogenic response in the nucleus.

Another reputed effect of PDGF is to activate the amiloride-sensitive sodium/ hydrogen ion exchange carrier. This system may be responsible for transducing mitogenic signals by processes that alkalinise the cytoplasm, with concomitant extrusion of hydrogen ions from the cell. An accumulation of all or some of these cellular effects elicits a mitogenic response in part by increasing cellular DNA synthesis.

Other cellular reactions of PDGF include increased lipid and protein synthesis, regulation of cellular receptor expression, e.g. those for transferrin, LDL and epithelial growth factor and facilitation of amino acid transport. Some of these actions may have a role in the overall mitogenic response of the cell. Although it also has to be remembered that PDGF has additional roles, including chemotaxis of monocytes and connective tissue cells, organisation of actin filaments of the cytoskeleton and stimulation of cell prostaglandin production.

PDGF AND THE CLINICIAN

If we recall that the biological action appears to be the proliferation of fibroblasts and smooth muscle cells, then there is one obvious major medical role for PDGF itself, and several for antagonists to it. The active role will probably be to promote wound repair, especially in situations where healing is poor, e.g. diabetic ulcers. Antagonists may be even more important, and in the era when proteins like PDGF can be produced by recombinant methods, it is equally possible to play around with nucleotide sequence to allow baterial expression of analogues which will act as competitive inhibitors. This might be important for the following:

(1) *Atherosclerosis.* This of course is an important cause of cardiovascular and cerebrovascular pathology and the involvement of lipids in this process has been described in Chap. 4a. However there is an important aspect to atherosclerosis outside lipids per se, namely the role of macrophages and monocytes which accumulate in the early fatty streak of the intima of the blood vessel, attracted there by a PDGF-like substance and interleukin-1 released from regenerating or damaged endothelium. This endothelial damage is probably exacerbated by toxic substances, such as oxidative components liberated from macrophages. Platelets adhere to the damaged endothelium, undergo the release-reaction and in so doing, release PDGF which then potentiates smooth muscle proliferation within the media of the blood vessel. These processes thus contribute to the atherosclerotic lesion. Inhibition is strongly to be desired.

(2) *Pulmonary fibrosis.* The fibrosis — a proliferation of smooth muscle cells and fibroblasts — caused for example by paraquat poisoning, which often results in death by respiratory failure might well be ameliorated by a PDGF antagonist.

(3) *Scleroderma.* There is enhanced fibroblast activity in scleroderma, a condition in which the skin becomes tough and leathery, and which probably has an autoimmune basis. Again a PDGF antagonist might prove helpful.

(4) *Arthridites.* There appears to be excess PDGF in synovial fluid in osteoarthritis, and enhanced PDGF receptors in chronic synovitis. The inflammatory process in such conditions must at least in part involve fibroblast proliferation. Again a designer antagonist might prove therapeutically valuable.

Further Reading

1. Holmsen H. Physiological functions of platelets. *Ann Med* **21** : 23–30, 1989.
2. Ross R. Platelet derived growth factor. *Lancet* **i**, 1179–1181, 1989.

PART FOUR

Defence Against Attack

18a
Lead

Presumably everybody now knows about the toxicity of lead subsequent to surmises about the Roman empire falling due to plumbism from its water pipes, and the disrepute of lead tetraethyl as an anti-knock agent in petrol. Lead (as villain) still crops up in surprising ways. It turns out that the Franklin expedition, which set off to survey the North West Passage in 1845, with two extremely well-fitted and provisioned ships, came awry because of lead poisoning. None of the explorers was ever seen alive again, and such clues as could be found in the Arctic wastes indicated mental confusion (the neuropathy of plumbism). The tobacco, tea and biscuits of the expedition were all wrapped in lead foil, and the canned food was exposed to a heavy seam of lead solder.

More recently, Dan Quayle has hypothesised that the thyroid conditions suffered simultaneously by Geoge Bush and his wife derived from the lead piping in the vice-presidential residence. He may be proved right if he goes the same way.

Nobody is now complacent about the possibility of lead toxicity. Most of us remain exposed to lead in the environment as unleaded petrol is still not mandatory in most countries and it has been shown that about 50% of the lead inhaled in car exhaust fumes can enter the bloodstream. In certain areas of the USA a 37% decrease in blood lead levels was observed when lead-free petrol was introduced. There is still lead piping in some water supplies. Even in a large city like Glasgow, up to 1977 the acidic, soft local water dissolved lead in the piping and gave the residents enhanced blood concentrations. The problem was reduced by replacing the lead pipes with alternative metals and also by reducing "plumb-solvency", that is increasing the pH and hardness of the water.

Children absorb about 40% of their oral intake of lead, as compared to about 7% in adults, so they are put even more at risk when playing in streets polluted by car exhaust fumes. Fortunately, lead-based paints (especially on toys!) are being phased out in most countries, reducing one more potential source of toxicity.

LEAD IN TISSUES

The bulk of absorbed lead is bound to the surface of red blood cells, only a small amount being free in plasma. Lead has been isolated from most tissues but an important site is bone where a large proportion can be stored as lead phosphate which replaces calcium phosphate in chronic lead exposure. The body finds it difficult to excrete lead and consequently it accumulates when there is persistent exposure. However some can be excreted in both urine and faeces.

CLINICAL MANIFESTATIONS OF LEAD TOXICITY

This problem is best considered from the point of view of short and long term exposure. In situations where acute exposure has occurred, such as cases of lead poisoning in demolition workers who were cutting up steel covered with lead paint, symptoms such as severe weakness and fatigue, abdominal pain, vomiting and nausea were in the forefront, along with sporadic constipation, anorexia and pleural pain. Long term exposure of workers in lead-related industries is thought to engender cerebral vasculature disease, extensor muscle weakness, peripheral neuropathy, and anaemia. Salient findings are the punctate basophilia seen on blood films of red cells and also the characteristic teeth staining lines in some victims of high, chronic, lead exposure.

DETECTION OF PLUMBISM

Blood is a suitable tissue for detecting lead toxicity not least because of its accessibility. It has been estimated that the half-life of lead in the blood is about one month, which may be misleading if the exposure is not continuous. Another possible problem is that upon very long-term lead exposure, as might occur over many years, some tissues such as bone become saturated such that their lead then becomes once again exchangeable with that of the blood; this has the effect of thus increasing the blood half-life to over a year in some cases. Further complexities result from the non-linear relationship between lead intake and blood lead; as the lead intake increases, the blood lead level increment gradually diminishes. Other complicating variables are increases in blood levels of smokers and the difficulty in interpretation of measurements in subjects of different ages.

At present there is controversy about acceptable lead intakes for populations. Studies in England showed that the daily lead intake is about 0.9 μmol, with 0.7 μmol being present in food sources, 0.1 umol in water and 0.1 μmol inhaled from the atmosphere; all these sources result in a median lead blood concentration of about 0.57 μmol/l. The World Health Organisation has considered a limit of 2 μmol/l in blood to be desirable. It has also been suggested that the maximum permissible level in expectant mothers and in children should be no more than 1.2 μmol/l. On an encouraging note, it appears that blood lead is gradually decreasing in UK populations, probably as a result of environmental policies instituted.

LEAD AND METABOLISM

The toxic effects of lead on living systems are mainly due to it binding to negatively charged chemical groups, such as carboxyl and sulphydryl functions in proteins. Consequently, it is not surprising to find it interfering with protein function and thus enzyme activity. For example, at concentrations of about 1.7 μmol/l in blood, red cell ATPase is inhibited.

At 2 μmol/l, peripheral neuropathy has been observed, with encephalopathy intervening at about double that figure. No less important is the possibility that exposure of children to lead can cause some degree of impaired intellectual performance. This is a highly controversial area, with divided opinions sometimes based on non-scientific perceptions; nevertheless it seems prudent to keep lead in the environment as low as possible.

Lead is known to inhibit various enzymes of haem synthesis (Fig. 45). The key enzymes are ferrochelatase and δ-aminolaevulinic acid dehydratase which are very sensitive to lead inhibition and as would be expected, inhibition of the dehydratase increases plasma and urine δ-aminolaevulinic acid whereas the inhibition of ferrochelatase causes an accumulation of protoporphyrin IX, the immediate precursor of haem in red cells. Because iron is less easily incorporated into the haem molecule as a result of ferochelatase inhibition, other metals are bound instead, such as zinc, thus zinc protoporphyrin is also a marker of lead intoxication.

MONITORING PATIENTS

Lead is now rather easily measured in blood and urine, the preferred method in hospital laboratories being atomic absorption spectrometry. However, blood and urine only reflect recent exposure and thus methods of assessing chronic toxicity are needed. Some scientists have advocated lead measurements in hair and teeth to provide an index of long-term exposure, but there are problems in standardising the sampling methods and in avoiding contamination. Certainly hair was informative in the case of John Torrington, a crew member in the Franklin expedition; it was 15 cm long, and sectioned transversely gave a temporal record of his exposure to lead throughout the voyage.

Another way of detecting lead intoxication is to measure the metabolites of porphyrin metabolism raised in red cells by inhibition of the enzymes catalysing haem synthesis (Fig. 45).

In summary, lead exposure is highly relevant to modern industrial, environmental and haematological medicine. It is moreover pertinent to public policy on waste disposal and pollution. The biochemistry laboratory can aid this complex via the detection and monitoring of subjects affected.

glycine + succinyl CoA

$\downarrow$ *δ-aminolaevulinate*
                    synthetase

δ-aminolaevulinate

$\downarrow$ *δ-aminolaevulinate dehydratase*

porphobilinogen

uroporphyrinogen I   uroporphyrinogen III

$\downarrow$ $\downarrow$

coproporphyrinogen I   coproporphyrinogen III

$\downarrow$

protoporphyrinogen IX

$\downarrow$

protoporphyrin IX

$\downarrow$ $\curvearrowleft$ Fe^{2+}

ferrochelatase

haem

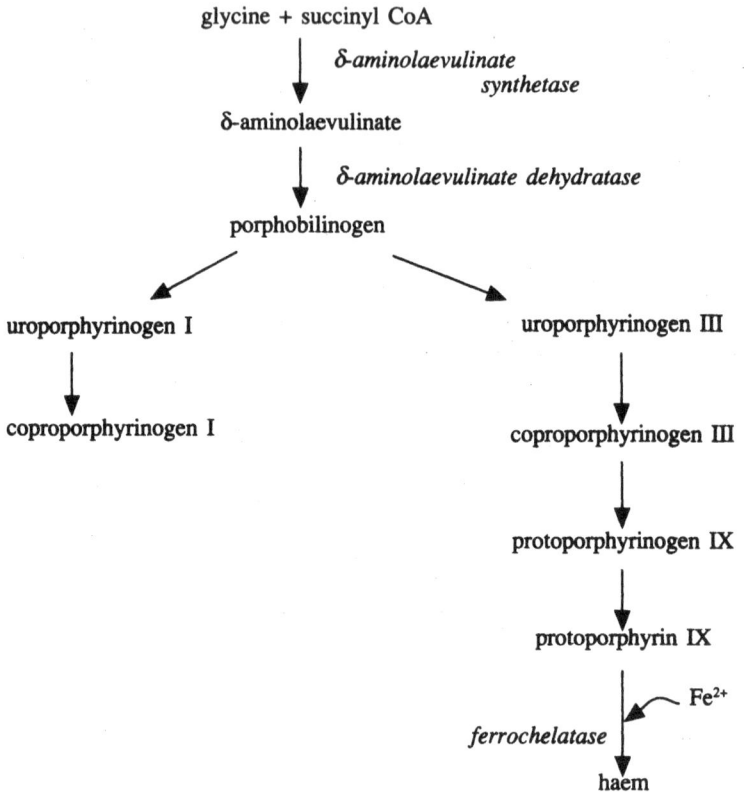

Fig. 45 A summary of porphyrin synthesis.

The rate-limiting step is the δ-aminolaevulinate synthetase. The other two enzymes shown, δ-aminolaevulinate dehydratase, and ferrochelatase, are the principal sites of interference by lead poisoning. At the branch point with porphobilinogen as substrate two interacting enzymes can form either uroporphyrinogen III or uroporphyrinogen I. The latter has no known physiological function, but may be formed in excess in some of the porphyrias. Uroporphyrinogen III represents the intermediate in the functional pathway.

Further Reading

1. Fell GS. Lead toxicity. *Ann Clin Biochem* **21** : 453–460, 1984.
2. Anon. Was the ill-fated Franklin expedition a victim of lead poisoning? *Nutr Rev* **47** : 322–333, 1989.

18b

Parkinsonism and Peroxidation

"The best thing about me now is my ear-lobes."
— the actor Terry Thomas, who died of parkinsonism

Parkinsonism is the term given to the syndrome consisting of tremor, hypokinesis (impairment of voluntary movement) and rigidity. In some parts of the Western world, the incidence is as high as 1% in people over the age of sixty years. The medical literature has recently revealed some fascinating new facets of this relatively common disorder, although it has to be said that its basic cause remains an enigma.

Radical Changes

In Chapter 16b, the imbalance between the neurotransmitters dopamine and acetylcholine in the substantia nigra of the brain was described as a factor in the pathogenesis of schizophrenia. Dopamine turns out have some connection with parkinsonism too, for some iatrogenic cases appear to be caused by dopamine blocking drugs. However the majority of cases are not drug-induced, in the sense of pharmacological drugs. Some substantive clues came from a few intravenous narcotics abusers who after injecting synthetic heroin showed features of chronic parkinsonism. Extensive biochemical and pharmacological detective work implicated a contaminant in the narcotic, a selective substantia nigral toxin named 1-methyl-4-phenyl-1,2,3,6 tetrahydropyridine, thankfully abbreviated to MPTP. This has the capacity to destroy dopamine containing neurones. Further work revealed that the toxin was not MPTP itself but a related compound MPP^+, or 1-methyl-4-phenyl-pyridinium, which blocks dopamine reuptake mechanisms. MPTP is a substrate for monoamine oxidase B, and is probably converted in the brain to MPP^+ via the intermediate compound methylphenyldihydropyridinium (MPDP) (Fig. 46). Indeed, the neurotoxicity of MPTP can be minimised by selective monoamine oxidase inhibitors such as deprenyl which blocks the conversion to MPP^+. Clearly, only very few patients with parkinsonian symptoms have abused contaminated synthetic narcotics but MPTP toxicity may form a working model for

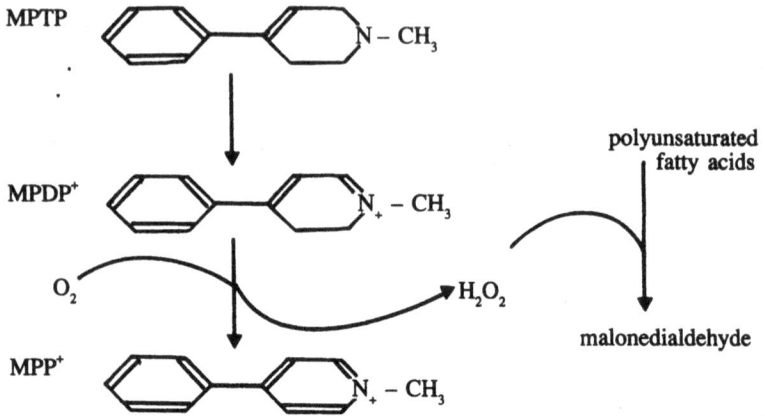

Fig. 46 The metabolic fate of 1-methyl-4-phenyl-1,2,3,6-tetrahydropyridine (MPTP).

MPTP, suspected as being implicated in Parkinson's disease, is a substrate for monoamine oxidase B (MAOB) and yields 1-methyl-4-phenyl-2,3-dihydropyridinium (MPDP⁺). A spontaneous oxidation gives the toxic 1-methyl-4-phenyl-pyridinium (MPP⁺) and the hydrogen peroxide thereby generated is noxious to the polyunsaturated fatty acids of neuronal membranes.

the mechanism of destruction of dopamine containing neurones.

MPP⁺ is chemically similar to the weed killer paraquat, a compound known to be important in free radical generation. Free radicals have cropped up repeatedly in these pages but once again we may note that they are chemical species with an unpaired electron, and are very reactive in that they attack molecules at positions of high electron density. Paraquat certainly exerts much of its toxic effect by generating free radicals in the lungs, causing necrosis, fibrosis and respiratory failure. Although MPP⁺ alone is unlikely to evoke free radical formation, in combination with MPDP⁺ a redox reaction occurs producing toxic superoxide radicals. It is these that are thought to be ultimately responsible for the neuronal damage. Some of the markers for cell death which might occur after free radical attack have been studied in brain tissue from parkinson sufferers — these are peroxidation products of polyunsaturated fatty acids, principally malondialdehyde. The results showed a decrease in substantia nigral polyunsaturated fatty acids and an increase in malondialdehyde, consistent with, though not necessarily proof of, a toxic free radical process taking place in this area of the parkinsonian brain. A candidate free radical is superoxide and it is of interest that the enzyme superoxide dismutase has been shown to be raised in the substantia nigra of patients with Parkinson's disease.

This enzyme catalyses the reaction which converts superoxide to oxygen and hydrogen peroxide in the presence of hydrogen ions

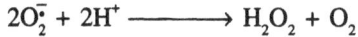

$$2O_2^- + 2H^+ \longrightarrow H_2O_2 + O_2$$

and may form part of a physiological protective system for inactivating free radicals. Why this enzyme is raised while other enzymes involved in protection against free radicals such as glutathione peroxidase are slightly decreased in Parkinson's disease is unclear but might reflect mitochondrial damage, since this peroxidase is largely mitochondrial. This latter suggestion would seem to have some foundation as the mitochondrial enzyme rotenone-sensitive NADH cytochrome c reductase, a component of mitochondrial complexes I and III has also been found to be reduced in this disorder.

At present one can only speculate on the mechanism of superoxide generation and subsequent mitochondrial malfunction, although some research has focussed upon the raised levels of iron in the substantia nigra also observed in Parkinson's disease — iron overload is another means of free radical generation. Whether this is a primary process or secondary to the disease is unclear. Substantia nigra ferritin, an important iron binding protein, has shown to be decreased in the disease.

CLINICAL OPTIONS

The research into MPTP has helped us gain an insight into some of the biochemical mechanisms in the brains of Parkinson's disease sufferers and has emphasised the concept of free radical involvement in disease states, but the basis of the disease itself remains obscure. Presumably, in the substantia nigra damage to dopamine rather than acetylcholine containing neurones takes place preferentially. The monoamine oxidase B inhibitor deprenyl (selegiline) slows the onset of parkinsonian disability, suggesting that free radical generating mechanisms similar to those involving MPTP but utilising intrinsic monoamines as substrates are important. Adjunct therapies may involve free radical scavengers such as vitamin E.

At least these manoeuvres are less drastic than the implantation of either autologous adrenal medullary tissue or heterologous foetal brain cells into the corpus striatum region of the brain of parkinsonian sufferers, with the idea of allowing the transplanted tissue to produce dopamine at the site of the brain deficiency.

Further Reading

1. Lunec J. Free radicals: their involvement in disease processes. *Ann Clin Biochem* **27** : 173–182, 1990.
2. Perry K. Neurotransmitters and diseases of the brain. *Br J Hosp Med* **45** : 73–83, 1991.

3. Williams A. Cell implantation in Parkinson's disease. *Br Med J* **301** : 301–302, 1990.

18c

Alcohol-related Disease: The Wrath of Grapes

ALL SYSTEMS GO

Quantitative estimates of the medical importance of alcohol-related problems vary, but all agree on their colossal magnitude. It seems, to take one simple statistic, that alcohol is involved one way or another in a third of all acute hospital admissions. On the pathophysiological side, it has been shown to affect every functional system, tissue, or cell so far examined. Here we abstract (1) cirrhosis of the liver; (2) the rate of clearance of alcohol from the blood in relation to police investigation of drinking and driving; and (3) the nutritionally-linked Wernicke-Korsakoff syndrome in order to relate basic biochemistry to interesting clinical areas.

Basically, the metabolism of alcohol is simple, if peculiar. It is metabolised to water and carbon dioxide (Fig. 47) but without any feedback controls, endocrine influences or membrane barriers. In fact it becomes completely distributed in the body water. Since in general women have a greater proportion of body fat than men, a given dose of alcohol tends to be more concentrated in their aqueous compartment, so they become drunk quicker (an observation which Sir Jasper and other evil squires made empirically; in fact, recent work has indicated that women have a less active alcohol oxidising system in the digestive tract itself, but the classical theory is by no means disproved.) Alcohol is an energy-yielding substance, the oxidation giving as much as 7 kcal/g, as compared to 9 kcal/g for fat, 4 kcal/g for carbohydrate, and 4 kcal/g for protein. About 90% of a bolus is metabolised by the liver, a consequence of the tissue distribution of the two enzymes which are immediately

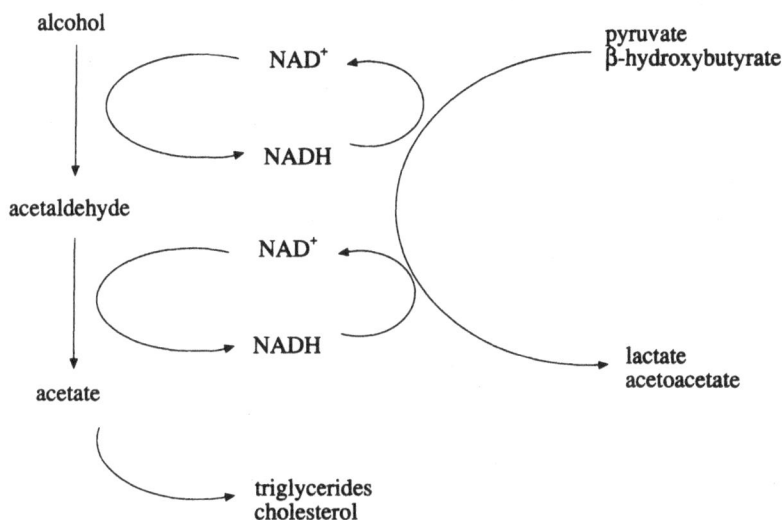

Fig. 47 Summary of alcohol metabolism.

Although many parts of the sequence are theoretically reversible, the arrows are all drawn in one direction to signify the disposal of a bolus of alcohol. In the presence of substrate the enzymes lactate dehydrogenase and β-hydroxybutyrate dehydrogenase dispose of the surge of NADH giving the corresponding reduced products. The acetate produced is a ready source of carbon atoms for lipid synthesis.

involved.

The one mole of acetic acid produced per mole ethanol ingested would cause a metabolic acidosis were it not readily assimilated for the synthesis of lipid and oxidation via the citric acid cycle. But the two dehydrogenases are non-specific and if methanol rather than ethanol is consumed then the end-product is formic acid, not readily metabolised, and causing a massive metabolic acidosis. Ethylene glycol, on the other hand, produces oxalic acid, which has the same effect. Since these substrates will all compete one with another for active site on the enzyme, it follows that you can decrease the conversion to formate and oxalate in poisoned individuals by persuading them to drink some whisky or brandy (beer is too dilute). As a first-aid measure, this may reduce the necessity for forced diuresis if there is admission to hospital as an emergency.

LIEBER'S BABOONS

There are three very broad aspects to alcoholic liver disease. The first is fatty infiltration, known as **steatosis**. The second is a necrotic process, or **alcoholic hepatitis**. The third, an irreversible change marked by massive deposition of collagen fibres, is considered to be a terminal, irreversible state and is known as cirrhosis. Taking these in turn:

(1) After alcohol ingestion, a plentiful supply of fat is potentially available due to the surge of acetate. It is well known from elementary biochemistry that all the carbon atoms of fatty acids and cholesterol may be derived from such two-carbon units. The fat so formed appears as large vacuoles in the hepatocyte, often flattening the nucleus against the cell membrane. Steatosis although found in a large number of alcoholics and thought to be a preliminary to more injurious changes is generally considered, in itself, to be benign and reversible.

(2) Obviously, an acute alcohol dose is first encountered by the liver at first pass and it may cause the hepatitic necrotic condition. It is established that alcohol causes a hypermetabolic state in the liver, for which all the oxygen demand is unlikely to be met. Comparative hypoxia causes plasma membrane damage, necrosis, and infiltration by polymorphonuclear leucocytes in an attempt, presumably, to remove the damaged cells. This of course constitutes an inflammatory process.

(3) Liver cirrhosis has been known for almost a century to be associated with alcoholism. Post-mortem or biopsy livers show focal necrosis and scar formation; this fibrosis distorts and compresses the regular structure of the lobules and acini. It may at length obstruct the portal vein, leading to portal hypertension, with ascites, as well as varicosities of the gastrointestinal tract veins. However, not all alcoholics become cirrhotic, and there is a puzzling international variation — in UK the prevalence of cirrhosis is one tenth that of France whereas the alcohol consumption is as much as one third of that country. In some experimental animals like rats, it cannot be produced at all, but C S Lieber fed alcohol to baboons for up to four years and found that all of them had fatty livers (thought to be an early stage in the pathological process) and a small proportion had frank cirrhosis.

What do we know of alcohol metabolism which can be linked to these fibrotic changes, which are considered to be the irreversible stage of alcoholic liver disease? First of all, disappearance of tissue through necrotic injury would in itself be expected to promote formation of scar tissue. But remember that above all else alcohol produces large quantitites of NADH, that is creates a reducing environment, hence the tendency to lactic acidosis and ketosis (Fig. 47). But further, formation of mature collagen requires the activity of proline hydroxylase, an enzyme utilising both oxygen and the hydrogen atoms/electrons from a reducing agent.

Thus the factors are in place — except that many alcoholics do not develop cirrhosis of the liver; so other agents are involved. But the same puzzling selectivity can be applied to many other diseases — cirrhosis of the liver is not alone in this respect. Statistics have been carefully gathered about alcoholic cirrhosis in different professions: in UK in 1990, the most prominent sufferers were, hardly surprisingly, publicans, with rates more than ten times the average. They were followed by seamen, barmen and managers in the entertainment industry. Reassuringly for our readers, nurses come bottom of the list, and doctors second bottom (somewhat below the clergy).

THE WERNICKE-KORSAKOFF SYNDROME

Two separate entities, Wernicke's encephalopathy and Korsakoff's psychosis are now usually conjoined as in the heading above, the former representing the acute, and the latter, the chronic phase of the disease. There is a tendency to call the condition **alcohol amnesic syndrome**, but this does not have the same resonance. It is a central nervous system condition characterised by ataxia, confusion and oculomotor disturbances, progressing to a chronic amnesia. It is primarily found in alcoholics (although it can also be a feature of stomach cancer, pyloric stenosis, vomiting in pregnancy, and total parenteral nutrition) and is rapidly cured, in the acute form at any rate, by massive doses of vitamin B1, thiamine. How does thiamine help? It is transformed in the liver to the coenzyme thiamine pyrophosphate (TPP), which is a coemzyme for at least three highly important reactions:

(1) Pyruvate dehydrogenase, in the entree to the citric acid cycle.

(2) α-ketoglutarate dehydrogenase, within the citric acid cycle.

(3) Transketolase, a prominent enzyme of the hexose monophosphate shunt.

If thiamine is missing in the diet, then the subject is obviously in trouble due to suboptimal substrate conversion in important pathways, and it is not surprising that this gives rise to a specific disease, beriberi. Alcoholics can have heart conditions related to beriberi, but Wernicke-Korsakoff is different because there is generally no lack of thiamine in their diet, rather one or more of their thiamine requiring enzymes is unable to bind TPP adequately.

We are familiar with inborn errors of metabolism due to missing enzymes, such as phenylalanine hydroxylase in phenylketonuria. Here, though, is another type of inborn error, whereby the enzyme is synthesised, and has potential catalytic function, but binds poorly to its coenzyme. Massive doses of the vitamin will however yield sufficient TPP to increase binding sufficiently (Fig. 48). The defect is also thought to be inherited. In the ordinary way, a non-alcoholic subject with the defect is protected by an adequate thiamine intake, an efficient absorption from the gastrointerstinal tract, as well as a competent conversion to the coenzyme form in

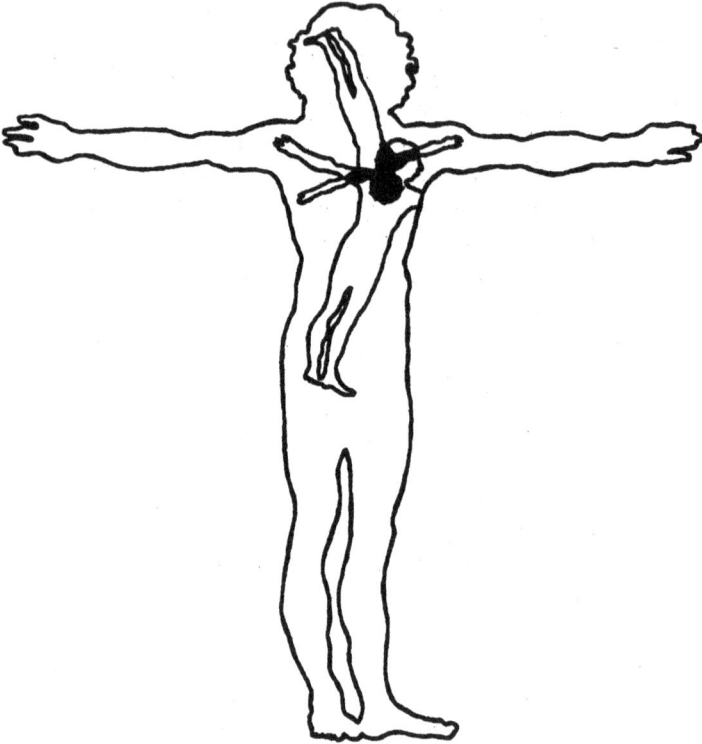

Fig. 48 Basis of the Wernicke-Korsakoff syndrome.

The large figure represents the total population under consideration, the intermediate figure those within it who, for whatever reason, become alcoholics, and the smallest those with a genetic defect in thiamine pyrophosphate binding to enzymes. The population which coincidentally suffers from both of these disabilities, represented by the shaded area, is prone to Wernicke-Korsakoff.

the liver. These last two are however compromised in the alcoholic and the psychosis may develop because there is just not enough thiamine available to produce a functional enzyme-coenzyme complex. It was shown directly in 1977 that the erythrocytic transketolase of subjects with the psychosis had deficient binding of TPP; of course, any connection between the diminished activity of enzymes 1–3 above and the CNS neuropathy remains obscure.

    There is an interesting clinical rider to all of this, in that if intravenous dextrose or other sugar-containing fluids are given to Wernicke-Korsakoff patients, their condition may actually deteriorate. This of course is because the load of carbohydrate produces large amounts of pyruvate which cannot be cleared in the absence of adequate amounts of TPP. The pyruvate produces lactate, and lactic acidosis is a serious and life-threatening condition in itself (Chap. 7a).

As a parting note to this topic, we may note that concerned authorities in many countries have tried to have all whisky and beer laced with thiamine by law. Well, already we buy water treated with fluoride, bread with calcium (and in some countries thiamine), salt with iodine, so the suggestion is not so novel. It turns out that some beers are more yeasty, therefore having more thiamine than others, so a nice controversy regarding consumer taste, the brewing industry, and public health has been rumbling on for some years, much to the entertainment of those with the time to follow it.

A BIOLOGICAL IMPOSSIBILITY

This is from a case reported by Professor Bernard Knight. In the early eighties, a prominent entertainer was caught speeding by the traffic police, and the breathalyser test being positive, he was taken to the station where he gave two samples of blood, one to be analysed in the Home Office Forensic Science Laboratory, which subsequently recorded a value of 31 mmol/l, the other given to the donor. Forty minutes later two more breath tests were performed to find if he was fit to return to his vehicle; they were both negative, implying a blood level of less than 18 mmol/l (in old units, 80 mg/100 ml, the legal limit). The subject had no chance to have the defence specimen analysed for ten days, but anyway at the end of that time, he was advised that an analysis was then not feasible due to deterioration of the analyte.

On coming to trial, the defence said that it was impossible for a person's blood to have 31 mmol/l alcohol at 7.26 p.m. and less than 18 mmol/l only 40 minutes later. Crucial to this advocacy is the known rate at which ethanol can be removed from the body. In effect there are three routes:
(1) Oxidation in the liver
(2) Expiration in the breath
(3) Filtration in the kidney
The last two are in effect minor mechanism, although they do contribute, and the overall rate was worked out in the thirties by Widmark. This is generally taken to be between 2.2 and 5.5 mmol/l (of whole blood) per hour (correct scientific notation $2.2-5$ mmol.l^{-1}.h^{-1}) The fall in concentration in the case of of the entertainer would have to have been 20 mmol .l^{-1} .h^{-1} which seems very high, Nonetheless the magistrates (this was not a trial by jury) convicted the defendant. At the appeal, the judges maintained that the prosecution need only show that at the time of the blood sample being taken the concentration was over 18 mmol/l, and the issue of impossibility was ducked. This might have been a happy decision (although Professor

Knight disagrees) for "impossible", like "never", is a word that one can regret using. A blood alcohol decay curve is seen in Fig. 49; it is a typical pharmacokinetic process, and the linear part is supposed to show a drop of 4 mol.l^{-1} .h^{-1}, on average. The range 2.2–5.5 is the group or population variance, which is normally computed as two standard deviations beyond the mean on both sides, and this mathematically covers 95% of the population under scrutiny, whatever that may be. So there have to be one or two people with very high or very low clearances way beyond the "normal range". A criminal tribunal gives a guilty verdict when satisfied "beyond reasonable doubt" and so apparently in this case it was content as to the accuracy of the first, blood alcohol determination. It is interesting to speculate, though, whether the magistrates understood, or even wished to understand, the issues as detailed above.

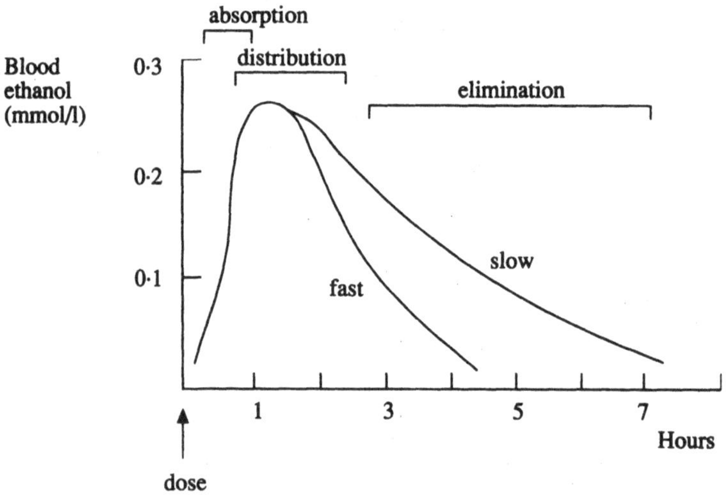

Fig. 49   Alcohol elimination chart.

Further Reading

1. Rosalski SB (ed). *Clinical Biochemistry of Alcoholism*. Edinburgh:Churchill Livingstone, 1984.
2. Knight B. Driving and alcohol: Case report of a biological impossibility. *Medicine, Science and the Law*, **24** : 271–273, 1984.
3. Geokas MC. Ethyl alcohol and disease. *Med Clin N Am* Jan 1984. Philaadelphia: Saunders, 1984.

18d

Ending Up and Aluminium

Aluminium is the third most abundant element (and the most abundant metal) in the Earth's crust so we are exposed to considerable amounts of it. Only recently has it become important in medicine.

RENAL DISEASE

In 1972 a syndrome was described in patients on long-term dialysis treatment. They exhibited a progressive and fatal neuropathy, termed dialysis encephalopathy syndrome, (DES). The symptoms of this condition were dramatic — confusion and speech impairment followed by convulsions, dementia and finally coma leading to death. In one large study in USA about 4% of dialysis patients manifested DES.

Initially, a variety of agents were implicated, but gradually it became evident that aluminium was the most likely candidate. This was based on animal studies in which similar symptoms were observed when they were given high aluminium diets, and also in human studies where it was shown that patients with DES had high brain and serum aluminium levels. In addition, areas in which the amount of aluminium in the drinking water is high, like Glasgow, were shown to have more DES than other areas. (The inhabitants of Glasgow were unlucky with their lead, too, Chap. 18b.)

How aluminium elicits DES, if indeed it is the culprit, is at present unclear, although some suggestions have been made. Some have proposed that it can reduce brain glucose uptake by inhibiting the enzyme hexokinase, others that it can decrease brain tetrahydrobiopterin by inhibiting the enzyme dihydropteridine reductase. Tetrahydrobiopterin is a cofactor for the synthesis of tyrosine from phenylalanine, and also (more significantly for brain) for the neurotransmitter serotonin.

Aluminium has also been implicated in other clinical conditions associated with renal disease. In dialysis/renal osteodystrophy, there appears to be normal magnesium and calcium balance but patients are relatively refractory to 1,25-dihydroxycholecalciferol therapy (as the active form of vitamin D) and also seem to present with more bone fractures. Despite some similarities to classical osteomalacia, in that there is unmineralised osteoid in the bone, the incidence of bone fractures in these patients is higher and they were shown to have very high tissue levels of aluminium. Aluminium would appear to alter the response of bone phosphatases to 1,25 dihydroxycholecalciferol and parathyroid hormone, resulting in reduced mineralisation.

Anaemia is common in renal failure and the normochromic, normocytic anaemia often described is probably partly the result of low erythropoietin production by the kidney itself (Chap. 13b). In contrast is the hypochromic, microcytic anaemia associated with high serum aluminium levels but normal serum iron, presumably yet another manifesation of the metal's toxicity. This type of anaemia may be due to inhibition of some enzymes of haem synthesis, such as uroporphyrinogen decarboxylase. Alternatively, aluminium may compete for iron binding to the iron transport protein transferrin.

An alarming suggestion is that sudden cardiac death in some renal dialysis patients may be the result of aluminium toxicity to the heart. This needs substantiation although it is known that aluminium can inhibit some cardiac enzyme systems involving ATP.

Why then is it that renal dialysis patients have this propensity towards aluminium toxicity and high serum aluminium concentrations? One possibility is that they tend to have elevated phosphate levels as a result of impaired renal excretion. Oral hypophosphataemic agents, binding phosphate in the intestine, have been used to treat hyperphosphataemia but many of them contain aluminium hydroxide, normally not absorbed from the intestine. It would seem that uraemic patients do have an increased intestinal absorption probably as a consequence of some abnormality of the gut wall. Another source of the elevated aluminium, before the problem was attacked by the formularists, was the dialysis fluid itself, which because of contamination, high aluminium water areas, or the use of aluminium salts as flocculants to remove organic material, was itself a cause of the loading.

As a result of these observations steps have now been made to reduce aluminium intake in renal dialysis patients through the use of alternatives to aluminium in phosphate binding agents and strict precautions in the preparation of dialysis fluids. It has been discovered that a dilaysis fluid pH of 7.0 will keep aluminium as water-insoluble aluminium hydroxide, and thus confined to the machine side of the dialysis membrane. For patients exhibiting raised body aluminium levels, the chelating agent desferrioxamine has been used.

Hopefully as a result of these procedures, aluminium toxicity in renal dialysis patients should be considerably reduced. To aid this, careful monitoring of serum aluminium is necessary. Care is needed to do this adequately as aluminium is present in glass and thus laboratory vessels. Aluminium has been shown to leach out of blood collection tubes resulting in contamination of the sample. However, if stringent care is paid this can be minimised, and aluminium measured accurately with atomic absorption spectrometry.

In terms of numbers of dementia patients, the role of aluminium in DES almost pales in comparison to Alzheimer's dementia.

ALZHEIMER'S DISEASE

The term dates from a description early this century of a progressive irreversible loss of memory, with apathy, deteriorating cognitive facilities, speech and gait defects, and disorientation. It is more common in women than in men, and is described as a presenile dementia, usually first occurring between the ages of 40 and 60. It is estimated to afflict about 5% of the population over 65, which works out to about two million people in the USA. In developed countries, as with any other disease of old age, it can only become quantitatively more important.

The brain shows characteristic changes at autopsy, with neuronal cell loss and the occurrence, throughout the cerbral cortex and the cerebellum, of the so-called senile plaques and neurofibrillary tangles. The plaques have extracellular deposits of A4 amyloid fibrils and these are associated with abnormal cholinergic nerve processes. The amyloid deposits themselves are derived from a protein called amyloid precusor protein, the gene for which is on chromosome 21.

When the characteristics of sufferers were studied, the two most important risk factors turned out to be age and family history. Age is bound to be a factor, by definition, but the genetics are obscure as sporadic cases with no evidence of family aggregation comprise a significant percentage of the whole, and moroever there is only a 50% concordance in identical twins. Other predisposing factors are a history of head trauma and thyroid disease. Senile plaques and neurofibrillary tangles invariably appear in Down syndrome patients, which again implicates chromosome 21, although not necessarily at the same locus as for amyloid precursor protein. Then there is aluminium. The evidence suggesting that aluminiun is implicated in Alzheimer's dementia is:

(1) Epidemiological data connecting incidence to aluminium in the water supply.
(2) High concentrations of aluminium in the plaques and tangles.
(3) Presence of amyloid precursor protein and A4 amyloid in renal failure patients with aluminium toxicity.
(4) Removing aluminium with the metal chelating drug desferrioxamine slows the rate of mental deterioration in a number of cases.

BIOCHEMICAL DIAGNOSIS OF ALZHEIMER'S DISEASE

It is important to be able to diagnose the disease accurately for if the dementia is *not* Alzheimer's then alternative causes may be successfully tackled. In some instances, brain biopsies have been performed — yes, seriously — but there is now some evidence that amyloid precusor protein is deposited systemically and we await a suitable method based on monoclonal antibodies to determine whether it is building up in the blood or skin. At the time of writing, though, there is no biochemical test or group of tests with sufficient specificity and sensitivity to be put into routine practice.

That being the case, the elimination tests are very important — glucose to eliminate hypoglycaemia, kidney function tests, serum electrolytes including calcium, thyroid function tests, and vitamin status (especially B_{12} and folate) and in addition, tests for syphilis and human immunodeficiency virus.

PARTING SHOTS

(1) It is as well to keep a watching brief on the quality of one's neighbourhood water. In July 1988, in Camelford, England, a crisis occurred when about 20 tons of 8% aluminium sulphate was accidently unloaded into the public drinking water supply. Aluminium was being used generally as a purifying agent because of its flocculating action upon particles. Many people who consumed this "polluted" water experienced unpleasant effects, such as abdominal symptoms.

(2) Is it likely, that a lifetime's exposure to aluminium is the basic cause of Alzheimer's — in other words, should we throw out all our aluminium cooking pans and kettles? Most of the authorities think this is premature, citing such items as the lack of increased risk of the disease among workers in aluminium smelters and bauxite mines. It seems more probable that the primary lesions in Alzheimer's damage the blood brain barrier in some way to allow an influx of aluminium, which then exerts its neurotoxic effects.

(3) The other common method of contact with aluminium is in the form of antacids which consist largely of aluminium hydroxide (sodium bicarbonate antacids of course contribute an unacceptable load of sodium to the system). They neutralise stomach hydrochloric acid to yield aluminium chloride and water. The chloride is thought to be passed staight through to the faeces, but who knows? At one time, it was thought that aluminium salts are not at all absorbed, but now it appears that this is not true, at least in subjects with renal impairment. As we grapple with the stresses of professional and family

life in middle age, and feel the gastric hydrochloric acid refluxing painfully up our oesophagi, and when we stretch out our hands for those aluminium antacids, are we not trading off gastritis against Alzheimer's? Which would we prefer? Or is the answer, rather, to make sure that one takes good care of one's kidneys?

Further Reading

1. Starkey BJ. Aluminium in renal disease. *Ann Clin Biochem* **24** : 337–344, 1987.
2. Katzman R and Saitoh T. Advances in Alzheimer's disease. *FASEB J* **5** : 278–286, 1991.
3. Sherrard DJ. Aluminium — much ado about something. *N Eng J Med* **324** : 558–559, 1991.

Index

A
Acetone 27
Acetylcholinesterase 9
Acidosis, metabolic 91, 163
       respiratory 162, 163
Acid phosphatase   14
Acne 71, 198
Acromegaly 141, 154
Actinin 4
Acute phase response 220
Addison's disease 158
Adenosine 52
Adriamycin 202
Ageusia 152
AIDS 43, 63, 218
Albumin 8, 29, 56, 178, 180, 220
Alcohol 34, 52, 53, 78, 93, 97, 144, 165, 191, 236
Alcoholic amnesia syndrome 239
Aldolase 3
Aldose reductase 32, 88
Alkaline phosphatase (AP) 14, 73
Alkalosis, metabolic   162, 163
    respiratory 163
Alphafoetoprotein 8, 13
Alzheimer's disease 20, 245
Aluminium 243
Amadori rearrangement 24
Amenorrhoea 128
Amniocentesis 9
Amyloid 17, 245
Anaemia 167
Androgens 72
Angioedema 152
Angiotensin 150
Angiotensin converting enzyme (ACE) inhibitors 149
Angiotensinogen 149
Anion gap 143, 164

Variable number tandem repeat (VNTR) 36
"Venuses" 132
Very low density lipoproteins (VLDL) 56, 109
Vitamin A 110, 130, 193, 198
Vitamin B1 (thiamine) 193
Vitamin B2 (riboflavin) 193
Vitamin B3 (nicotinamide) 193
Vitamin B6 193
Vitamin B12 (cobalamin) 193
"Vitamin B15" 192
Vitamin C 184, 202
Vitamin D 79, 87, 110, 154, 193, 243
Vitamin E 186, 193, 202, 235
Vitamin K 193
Vomiting 161, 206, 230
von-Gierke's disease 54, 94

W
Wernicke-Korsakoff syndrome 236
Werner's syndrome 121
Wound healing 217

X
Xanthine 52
Xanthomas 56, 148
Xerophthalmia 197

www.ingramcontent.com/pod-product-compliance
Lightning Source LLC
Chambersburg PA
CBHW061240220326
41599CB00028B/5489